THE Illustrated
MATERIA MEDICA

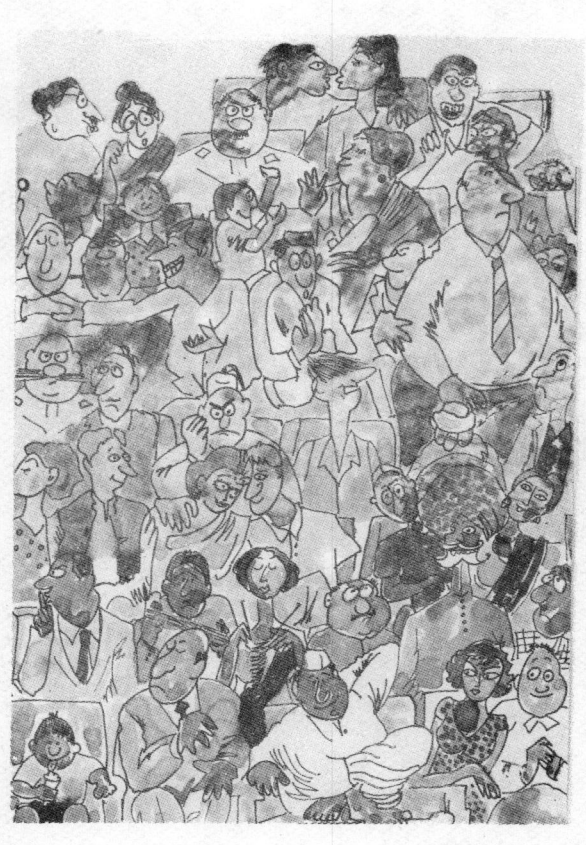

THE
ILLUSTRATED
MATERIA MEDICA

Dr. Kamal Kansal
D.H.M.S., M.F. (Hom.)
Gold Medalist

Foreword by

Dr. Diwan Harish Chand

B. JAIN PUBLISHERS (P) LTD.
An ISO 9001 : 2000 Certified Company
USA — EUROPE — INDIA

THE ILLUSTRATED MATERIA MEDICA

First Edition: 1981

Second Edition: 1990

Third Revised & Enlarged Edition: 1994

Reprint Edition: 1998, 2000, 2007

Published by Kuldeep Jain for
B. Jain Publishers (P) Ltd.
An ISO 9001 : 2000 Certified Company
USA — EUROPE — INDIA
1921, Street No. 10, Chuna Mandi,
Paharganj, New Delhi 110 055 (INDIA)
Phones: 91-11- 2358 0800, 2358 1100, 2358 1300
Fax: 91-11-2358 0471; *Email:* bjain@vsnl.com
Website: **www.bjainbooks.com**

Printed in India by
J.J. Offset Printers
522, FIE, Patpar Ganj, Delhi - 110 092
Phones: 91-11-2216 9633, 2215 6128

ISBN: 978-81-319-0053-6
BOOK CODE: 0053

FOREWORD

It gives me pleasure to write a foreword to "The Illustrated Materia Medica" written by my young colleague Dr. Kamal Kansal who was previously my student.

What fascinates me specially are the cartoon pictures that illustrate the symptoms of the remedies. Such visual impressions are computerised in our brain much better and leave a more lasting impression available for later racall than mere reading of written text. The study and memorising of Homoeopathic Materia Medica is a very diffcult thing and any aid to it is most welcome.

I am tempted to reproduce from the introduction of another similar book.

"There are two clearly defined schools of thought regard to the amassing and retaining of data."

The more Spartan school believes in sitting up to a table on a hard chair and squarting up to the job, and the followers of this school say with some justice that what is learned the hard way is better remembered, and a distinguished educationlist, in discussing the possibilities of education by the cinema, uttered the dictum that "Peptonised mental pabulum atrophies the intellectual digestion."

All this may be true paticularly when applied to sequential science which can be developed logically from first principles.......but on the other hand where we come to the memorising of isolated facts which can not be arrived at by a chain of reasoning, we are presented with the alternatives of either learning them parrot-wise with much effort, or of forming some memory associations which will present us with at least a starting point. I would most certainly opt for the second method and I think given the choice who would not. I have therefore consistently advocated and followed audiovisual methods in teaching my students.

The chief value of this book is to aid the students to master that which is guiding and characteristic in the individuality of some important remedies by way of illustration. It is by no means meant to be a comprehensive materia medica or an exhaustive study of the remedies considered.

I trust that the book will be welcomed not only by the students but also by the teachers as an aid to teaching and by the practitioners as a refresher and interesting study.

1, Hanuman Road
New Delhi - 110 001
October, 1981

DIWAN HARISH CHAND

PREFACE TO THE FIRST EDITION

This book is an attempt to provide a concise yet reasonably complete, uptodate review of difficult subject for use by Homoeopathic students and general practitioners.

My idea for presenting this book to the Homoeopathic fraternity is to put it into a comprehensive format to encompass the charcteristics and leading symptoms of the polychrest remedies so as to make the way easy for understanding and remembering the Materia Medica, the bedrock of Homoeopathy.

I hope it will serve the readers as companion volume to the standard texts as well as a quick reference guide. The readers will find this work as an accompaniment from which to seek out the more extensive texts for additional information necessary to a fuller understanding of this difficult speciality.

Out of the detailed text, not all the symptoms are important. The leading and striking symptoms of a particular drug are usually few on which homoeopathic prescribing often depend. So the purpose of these illustrations is to place a graphic portrait of the selections in this compilation in such a way that a basic posture of the remedy may be retained easily and permanently in the mind.

I believe that the multiplicity and magnitudes of symptomatology recorded under a drug by various authors is more of a deterrent in absorbing the spirit and individuality of a drug, thus, making the study of Materia Medica least interesting. The effort is to generate and instinctive affinity and inerest in making its understanding easier, likeable and interesting.

The reader who finds these illustraions of some use in memorising the drug picture should try his imagination to illustrate his own favourite remedies pertaining to his own memory problems.

I place on record my gratitude to all my colleagues who extended all the help and cooperation in making this venture a success.

I am sincerely grateful to Dr. Diwan Harish Chand for having written the Foreword and for his encouraging comments.

I am indebted to Mr. Kapil Kansal for his patience and fine work in making the drawings convey the ideas I have to stress. Also, I wish to thank Mr. Rajwansh Prasad for his untiring work in typing the manuscript as it was being produced.

New Delhi   **KAMAL KANSAL**
October, 1981

PREFACE TO THE SECOND EDITION

When this work was published in 1981, it was assumed that this will provide the homoeopathic student an easy tool to memorize salient characteristics of important homoeopathic remedies but, it is gratifying, that it received equally flattering reception from homoeopathic teachers and physicians as well. It was a matter of time that thousand odd copies which were printed got exhausted. Although the second edition should have been published some four years back, it could not be so because of some pressing preoccupation.

This edition is thouroughly revised and rearranged removing the errors which had crept in inadvertantly in the earlier edition. Besides, eight new remedies have been included in this edition.

It is hoped that this edition shall receive such reception and reviews as were received by the earlier edition.

New Delhi   **Kamal Kansal**
January, 1990

PREFACE TO THE THIRD EDITION

This third edition is new, the text is rewritten and illustrations redrawn. The source and preperation of the drug is equally important, this is one among other new features. The entire symptomatology of a drug gives a clear indication of it's origin either one or many, this is nothing but the pathogenetic sphere of action of that particular drug e.g. the pain of Bryonia in knee, chest, every where worse by least movement is because of its effect on serous membrane or nausea, retching with cough in Ipecac or Ant. tart is owing to their effect on Vagus, so on and soforth, this is also a new feature this time.

Text that mean the salient symptoms are in bigger type same as were in earliar editions with additions ofcourse. Homoeopathic prescription revolves around modification of a situation - how and what modifies ? Is it not strange, bacterias harbouring in the throat attacks only on one tonsil either Rt or Lt. at one time, pain of gout or arthritis are better by rubbing ice, or toothache is better by smoking ? This peculariity is unique with homoeopathic prescription - after all every individual is individual .

Dosage remains neglected topic and leaves the prescription incomplete. Most of the potencies and dosages are, what I have been using and found many thousand times clinically verified. But nothing is best than your own experience. However to start with 30th is advisable.

I am thankful to Miss Kalpana for having drawn all the illustrations in the manner they are required to portray the symptoms , making them more catching and memorable, Dr. Babita for her kind help in collecting the details for revised text, to the staff at M/s grafikman advertising agency for their co-operative attitude, and M/s B. Jain publishers for kindly publishing it.

I am once again sure that this new revised and enlarged edition would receive much more flattering reception from homoeopathic fraternity.

New Delhi   **Kamal Kansal**
20th August, 1994

CONTENTS

To
my teachers, past, present and future
this book is gratefully dedicated

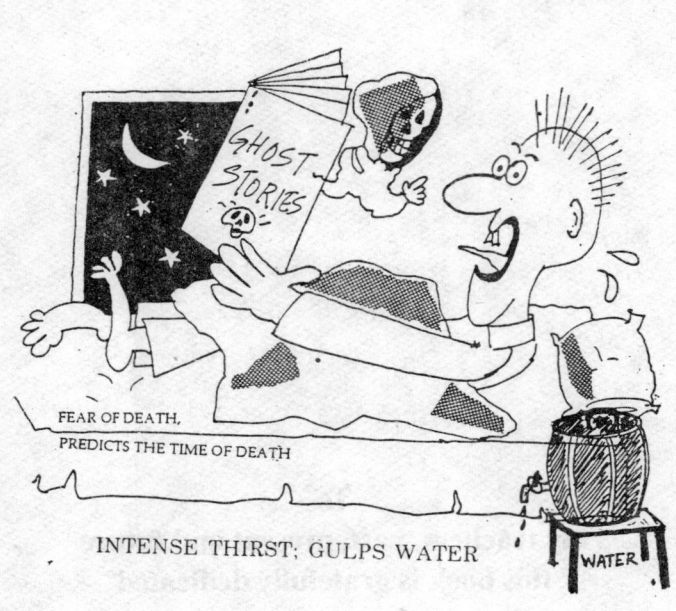

FEAR OF DEATH,
PREDICTS THE TIME OF DEATH

INTENSE THIRST; GULPS WATER

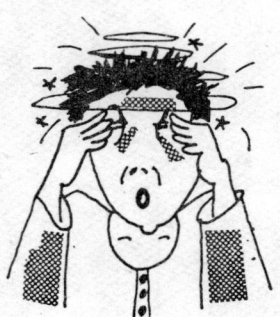

BURSTING HEADACHE & VERTIGO WORSE
ON RISING AND SHAKING HEA.

ACONITUM NAPELLUS

Commonly called Aconite. Common name Monkshood, wolfsbane N.O. Ranunculacae. Tinchure of whole plant with root when beginning to flower is used.

Pathogenetic sphere of action:
- The circulatory system: congestion with possible hypertension, flushing of face. Possibility of artirial haemorrhage is always very high.
- The nervous system: Causing excitement, anxiety, restlessness, fear in general and particularly fear of death.
- Intense neuralgic phenomena in Trigemial area.

Marked physical and mental restlessness.

Fright, delirium, thirst, fever and anxiety.

Acute, sudden and violent invasion with fever after exposure to dry cold weather.

Fears death; predicts the day and the hour of death.

Fullness and heat in head. Bursting headache; vertigo; worse on rising.

Ear sensitive to noises; music is unbearable.

Smelling power acutely sensitive, dry coryza.

Face flushed, hot or becomes deathly pale on left side.

Tongue inflamed. Tonsils red and swollen. Bitter taste of everything except water.

Great thirst for cold water.

Oppressed breathing,dry cough; worse night.

Tachycardia,palpitation with anxiety,pulse full, hard, tense, bounding.

Bruised pain in back.

Numbness and tingling in extremities. Hot hands and cold feet.

Anxious dreams with restlessness.

Hot dry skin.

Fever - thirst, restlessness and mental anxiety.

Children fretful, always crying with convulsive disorders during teething.

Modalities: worse in warm room, evening and night, lying on affected side, from music, tobacco smoke, dry cold winds, sun heat. Better in open air.

Dosage: Almost all problems are associated with mental anxiety and restlessness, 200 few doses.

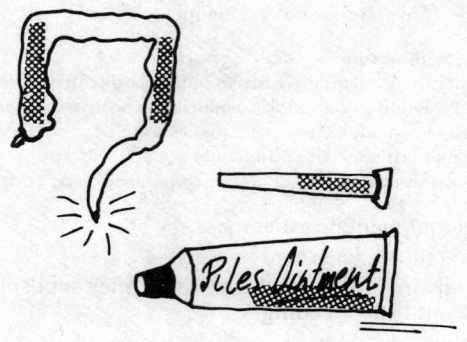

HAEMORRHOIDS; BLIND OR BLEEDING

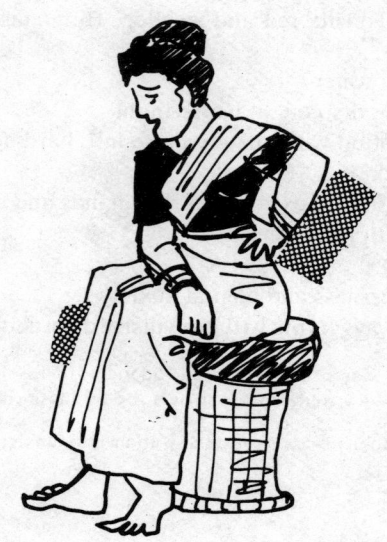

LUMBOSACRAL BACKACHE, WORSE WALKING AND STOOPING

AESCULUS HIPPOCASTANUM

Common name - Horse Chestnut. N.O. Sapiridacae. Tincture of ripe kernel, trituration of dry kernel or tinture of fruit with capsule is used.

Pathogenetic sphere of action:
-        Venous circulation causing; general plethora special action on portal and hepatic circulations. With important consequences upon haemorrhages and congestion of all the pelvic organs.
-        Lumbar spine; causing pains localized in the sacro iliac joints.
-        Mucous membranes; causing dryness, congestion esp. of mouth, throat and rectum.

Torpor and congestion of liver and portal system with constipation.
The back aches and gives out and unfits the patient for business.
Piles; Much pain but little bleeding.
Flying pains all over.
Fullness in various parts, dry, swollen mucous membranes.
Throat disorders with haemorrhoidal conditions.
Haemorrhoids with sharp shooting pains up the back, blind and bleeding.
Burning in anus with chills up and down back.
Region of spine feels weak, back and legs gives out, backache affecting sacrum and hips.

Modalities: Worse in morning on waking, motion, walking, eating after, standing. Better cool open air, soft easy stool.

Dosage: 30 potency 3 times, (needs some time to show action).

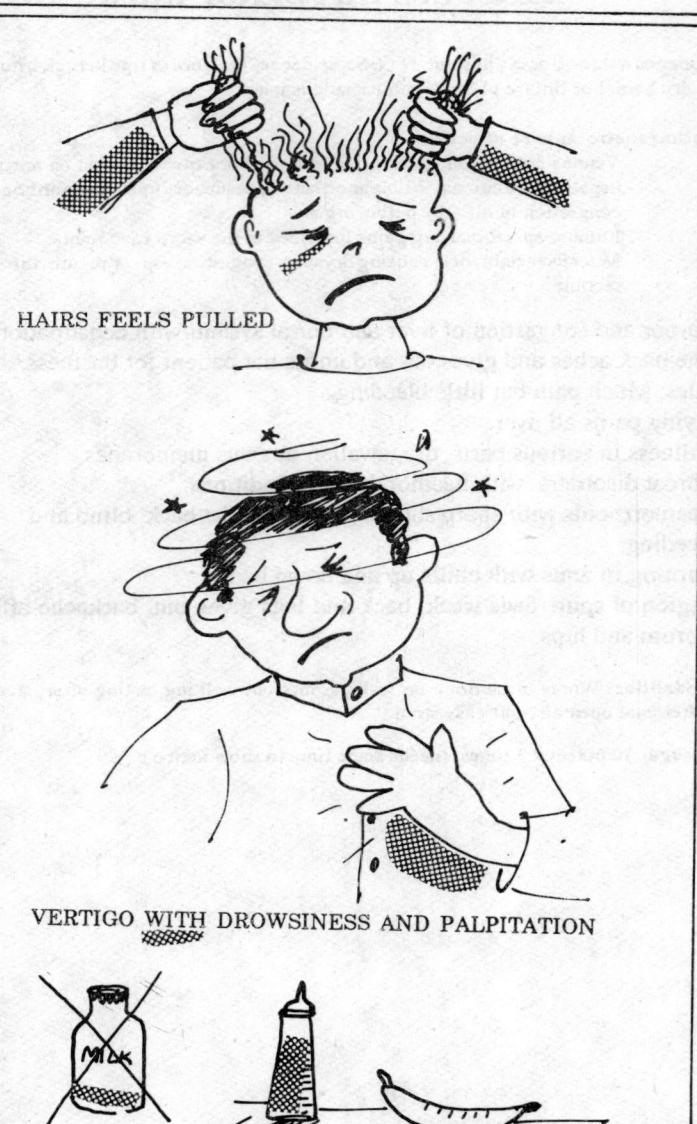

HAIRS FEELS PULLED

VERTIGO WITH DROWSINESS AND PALPITATION

INTOLERENCE OF MILK

AETHUSA CYNAPIUM

Fool's parsley N.O. Umbelliferae. Tincture of whole flowering plant

Pathogenetic sphere of action:
- The digestive system; causing severe vomiting and profuse diarrhoea. Intolerance of milk.
- The nervous system causing restlessness, and convulsions.

Anguish, crying and expression of uneasiness and discontent.

Disease of children during dentition, summer complaints.

With diarohoea there is marked inability to digest milk and poor circulation.

Symptoms set in with violence.

Inability to think, to fix the attention.

Eyes drawn downward pupil dilated.

Herpetic eruption on tip of nose.

Face puffed, red spotted, collapsed, linea nasalis marked.

Intolerance of milk vomiting as soon as swallowed.

Regurgitation of food about an hour after eating.

Vomiting with great weakness and sweat.

Stools are undigested, thin, greenish, preceded by colic with tenesmus and followed by exhaustion.

Surface of body cold and covered with clammy sweat.

Itching eruption around joints.

Child is so exhausted it falls asleep at once.

Modalities: Worse: 3 to 4 a.m., and evenings, summer heat, milk. Better in open air and company.

Dosage: 6th to be repeated often in acute gastro-enteritis complaint.
200 infrequently for cerebral symptoms.

F.2

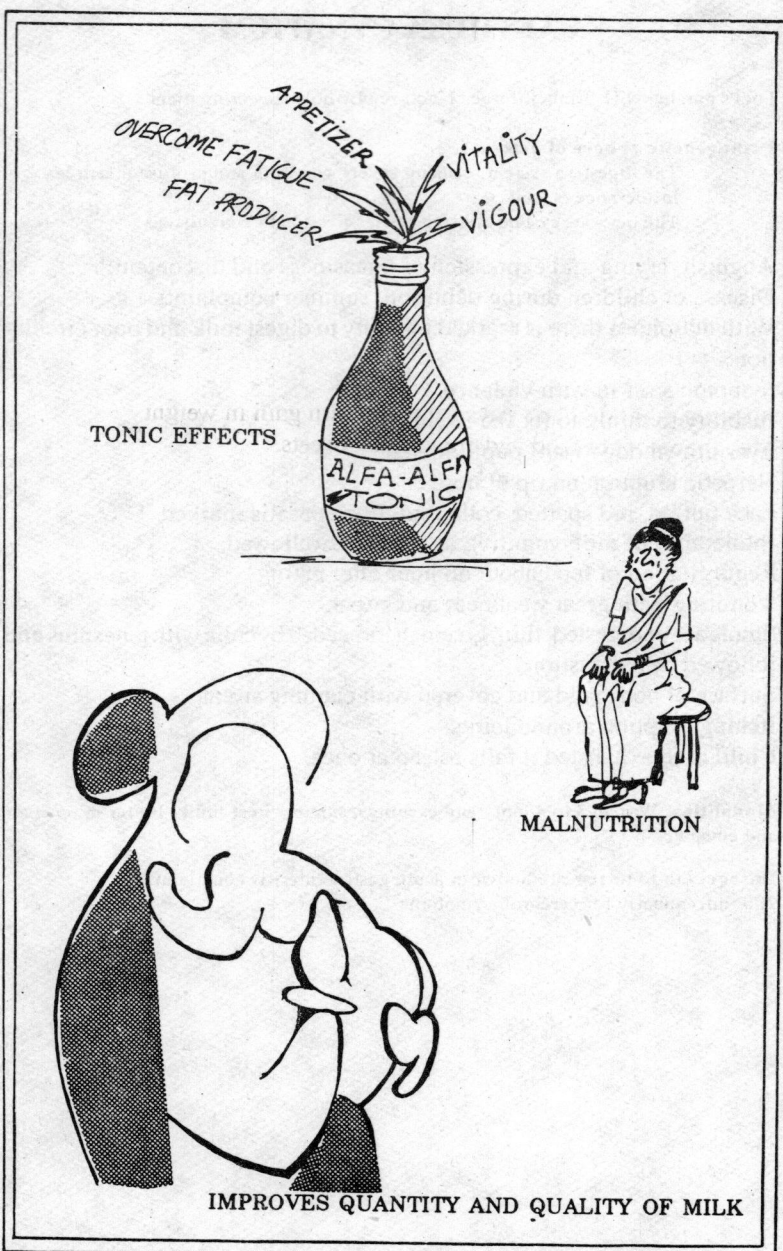

APPETIZER

OVERCOME FATIGUE

VITALITY

FAT PRODUCER

VIGOUR

TONIC EFFECTS

ALFA-ALFA
TONIC

MALNUTRITION

IMPROVES QUANTITY AND QUALITY OF MILK

ALFALFA

Califormia cloner or luceme. Tincture of whole grass shoot is used.

Pathogenetic sphere of action
- Digestive system enhancing appetite, assimilation and absorption of food.
- Nervous system, improving neurasthenia, nervousness, insomnia, consequent to mal-nutrition.
- Improves deficient lactation; increasing quality and quantity of milk in nursing mother, again if due to malnutrition.

It influencs nutrition, tones up the appetite, and digestion.

Deficient lactation, increases quality and quantity of milk in nursing mother.

It improves mental and physical vigor with gain in weight.

Much nibbling of food and craving for sweets.

Kidneys inactive, frequent urging to urinate.

Increased elimination of urea, indican and phosphates.

Modalities: Worse: Physical and mental exertion.

Dosages: Tincture 1Drops/10Kg. of weight. 3-4 times daily before meals. (Continue till its effects are appreciated).

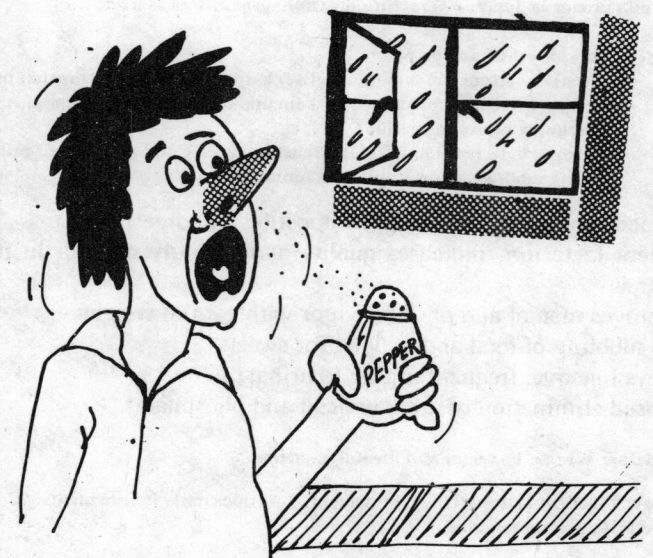

VIOLENT ATTACK OF SNEEZING WITH COPIOUS,
ACRID DISCHARGE WORSE IN WARM, CLOSE ROOM.

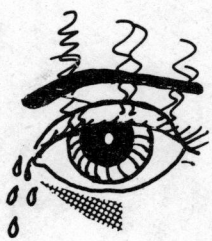

PROFUSE BLAND LACHRYMATION

ALLIUM CEPA

Common name Red onion N.O. liliacecae. Tincture of onion or of whole fresh plant gathered from July to August.

Pathogenetic sphere of action
- The upper respiratory mucosa and conjuctivae where it produces catarrhal irritation.
- The intestine causing flatulent colic.
- The sensory nervous system producing painful inflammation (facial nerves, damaged or sectioned nerves)

Profuse coryza with acrid nasal and bland eye discharges.

Catarrhal headache, worse in warm room and towards evening.

Eyes red, with much burning; profuse bland lachrymation; better in open air, burning eyelids.

Sneezing, especially when entering a warm room, profuse, watery, extremely acrid nasal discharge.

Hoarseness. hacking cough on inspiring cold air with tickling in larynx.

Sensation as if larynx is split or torn.

Oppressed breathing from pressure in the middle of chest.

Facial paralysis (Bell's palsy) of left side.

Pain in ear, shooting in eustachian tube.

Strong craving for raw onions. Cannot take any other nourishment.

Traumatic neuritis, often met within a stump after amputation.

Phantom limb sensation.

Modalities: Worse in evening, in warm room. Better in open air, in Cold room.

Dosage : 30th 3-4 times daily for rhinitis. 1M or above for neuralgias and neuritis.

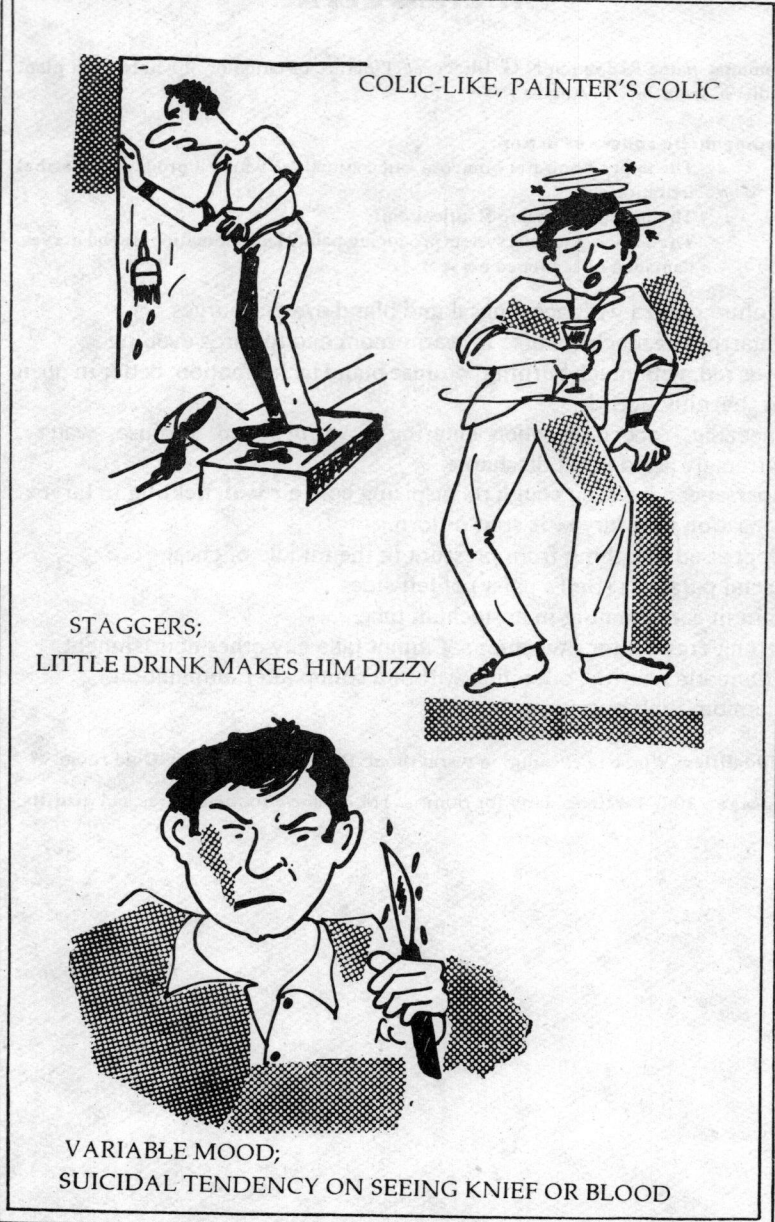

COLIC-LIKE, PAINTER'S COLIC

STAGGERS;
LITTLE DRINK MAKES HIM DIZZY

VARIABLE MOOD;
SUICIDAL TENDENCY ON SEEING KNIEF OR BLOOD

ALUMINA

Argilla oxide of Aluminium. Pure clay Al_2O_3 $3H_2O$ Trituration.

Pathogenetic sphere of action
- The skin and mucosa causing extreme dryness which secretes thick yellow mucus which is very difficult to remove.
- There is general paretic weakness and intestinal paresis causing constipation.

Complete dryness of mucous membranes, skin and tendency to paretic muscular states.

Mentally low spirited; fear, loss of reason. Hasty, hurried, time passes slowly, variable mood.

Suicidal tendency when seeing knife or blood.

Throbbing headache with constipation.

Abnormal cravings- chalk, charcoal, dry food etc.

Aversion to meat. Potatoes disagree.

Painter's colic. Left sided abdominal complaints.

Stool- hard, dry,knotty; no desire. Has to strain a lot, even for soft stool.

Must strain at stool in order to urinate.

Leucorrhoea acrid, profuse, transparent, ropy, worse during day time and after menses.

Menses too early, short, scanty, followed by great weakness.

Paralytic weakness in back.

Extremities feels weak and paralyzed.

Staggers on walking, little drink makes him dizzy.

Skin chapped, dry, intorlerable itching when getting warm in bed.

Sweat is rare and scanty.

Nails brittle.

Modalities: Worse periodically, in afternoon, from potatoes, in morning on waking, warm room. Better in open air, cold washing, in evening, alternate days, damp weather.

Dosage : 30th. Higher in Paralytic complaints.

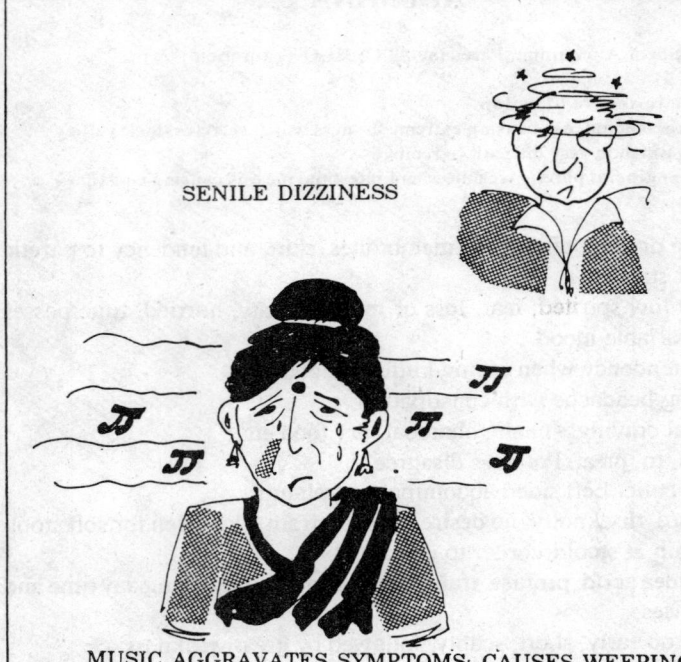

SENILE DIZZINESS

MUSIC AGGRAVATES SYMPTOMS; CAUSES WEEPING

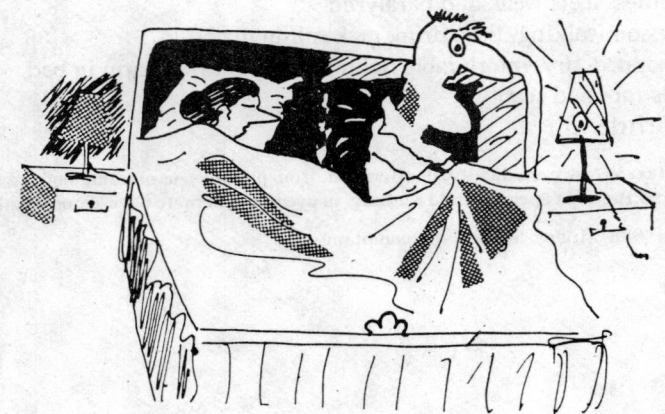

SLEEPLESSNESS DUE TO WORRIES; MUST GET UP

AMBRA GRISEA

Ambergris, It is a Morbid product found in the sperm whale or floating in the sea. Trituration and tincture.

Pathogenetic sphere of action.
- The nervous system causing sensitivity.
- The circulatory system causing capillary fragility with haemorrhagic tendencies.

There is extreme nervous hypersensitiveness.

For patients weakened by age or overwork.

There is weakness, coldness, numbness usuallly of single parts, fingers, arms etc.

Music aggravates symptoms. causing weeping.

Tearing pain in upper half of brain.

Senile dizziness.

Hearing is Impaired.

Distention of stomach and abdomen after midnight.

Feeling in urethra as if a few drops passed out.

Urine turbid even during emission forming a brown sediment.

Itching of pudendum with soreness and swelling.

Discharge of blood between periods, at every little accident.

Nervous spasmodic cough. With hoarseness and eructation on waking in morning, worse in presence of people.

Hollow spasmodic barking cough, coming from deep in Chest.

Palpitation with pressure in chest as from a lump lodged there, as if chest were obstructed.

Cannot sleep from worry must get up.

Cramps in hands and fingers worse grasping anything.

Modalities: Worse music, presence of strangers, from any unusual thing, morning, warm room.Better slow motion, in open air, lying on painful part, cold drinks.

Dosage : 3x for cough. 30th or higher for other complaints.

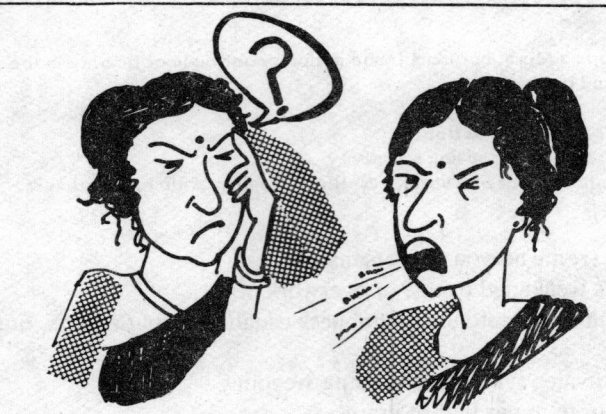

IMPAIRED MEMORY AND
ABSENT-MINDEDNESS

DESIRE TO CURSE AND
SWEAR AND TENDENCY
TO USE FOUL LANGUAGE

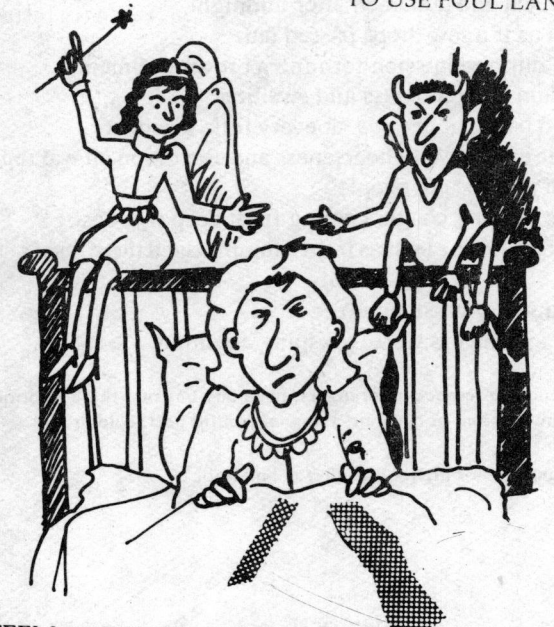

FEELS: A DEMON SITTING ON ONE SHOULDER AND ANGEL
ON THE OTHER (THINKS SHE IS POSSESSED OF TWO
PERSONS OR WILLS)

ANACARDIUM ORIENTALE

Commonly called Anacardium orientale. Common name Marking Nut N.O. Anacardiaceae. Trituration of layer of nut between shell and kernel.

Pathogenetic: sphere of action
- The nervous systems causing depression, loss of memory etc.
- The stomach.
- The skin causing vesico-pustular or phlyctenular eruptions.

Impaired memory. Absent-mindedness.

Low-spirited, disheartened, fears he is pursued, fears everything and everybody.

Morose, sulky, sullen.

Unsocial; irresistible desire to curse and swear; cruel, malicious, wicked. Very easily offended.

Hallucination: a demon sits on one shoulder and an angel on the other. "Feels as though he had two wills".

Pressing pain in head, as from a plug. Headache better during a meal.

Sensations of plug and also of a band in various parts of body as in rectum, throat etc.

Empty feelings in stomach, relieved by eating.

Ineffectual desire; rectum seems powerless, as if plugged up.

Hears voices from Heaven and Hell.

Intense itching; eczema; vesicular eruptions.

Full of trembling and paralytic weakness.

Tetanus.2

Epilepsy.

Modalities: Worse on application of hot water Better from eating, When lying on side, from rubbing.

Dosage : 12th 3 times a day.

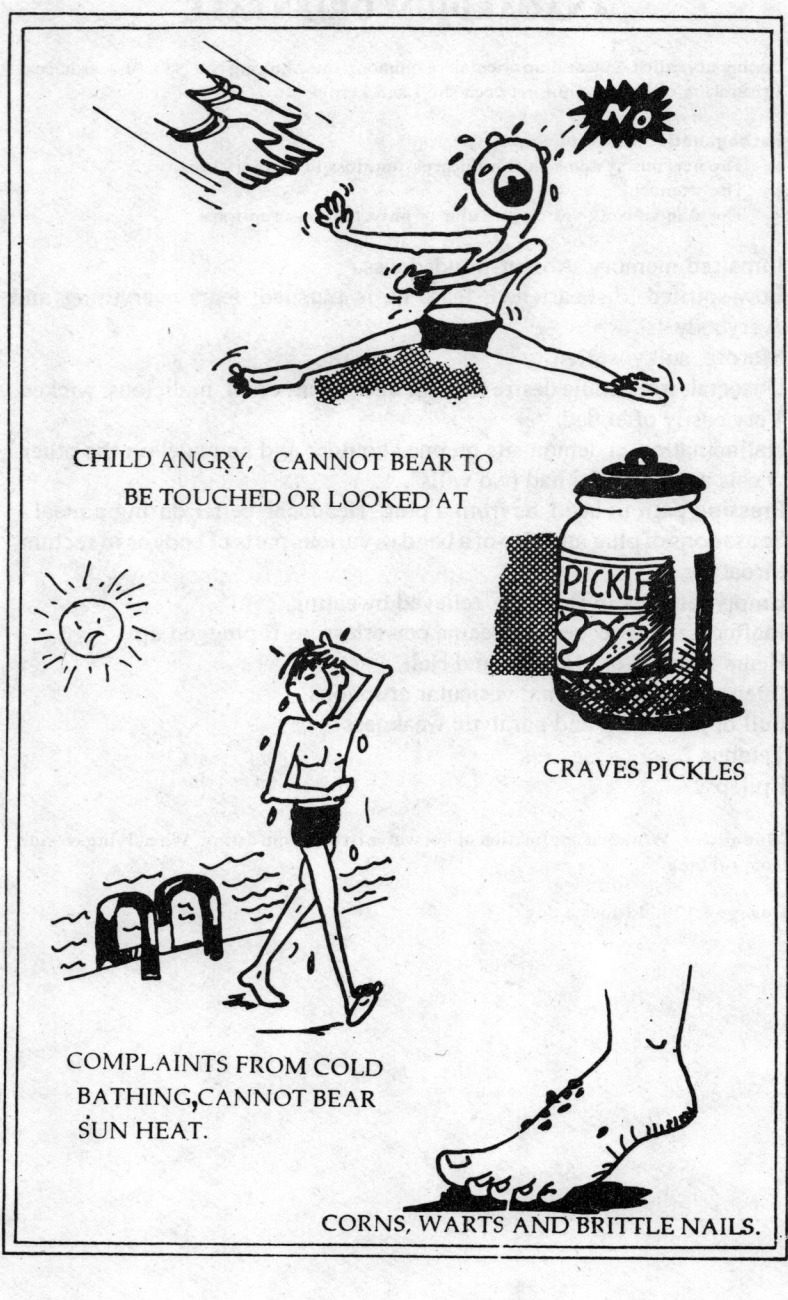

CHILD ANGRY, CANNOT BEAR TO
BE TOUCHED OR LOOKED AT

CRAVES PICKLES

COMPLAINTS FROM COLD
BATHING, CANNOT BEAR
SUN HEAT.

CORNS, WARTS AND BRITTLE NAILS.

ANTIMONIUM CRUDUM

Native sulphide of Antimony Sb_2S_3.

Pathogenetic sphere of action
- The digestive tract particularly the stomach.
- The skin.

Excessive irritability and fretfulness.

Child cannot bear to be touched or looked at. Sentimental mood in moon light. Abscence of the desire to live.

Headache from sun bathing or from disordered stomach, especially from eating candy or drinking acid wines etc.

Eyes agglutinated. corners fissured and raw.

Nostrils raw and ulcerated.

Cracks in the corners of mouth.

Tongue coated thick, white, as if white washed.

Loss of appetite. Desire for acid, pickles.

Eructations of ingesta. Vomiting of milk in curd form after nursing.

Constant belching and bloating after eating.

Diarrhoea after overeating, bathing in sun and from wines etc.

Continued oozing of mucus from anus, mucous piles.

Nails brittle, inflamed corns, pain in heels.

Continual drowsiness in old people.

Modalities: Worse in evening, from heat, acids, wine, water, and washing, wet poultices. Better open air, during rest, moist warmth.

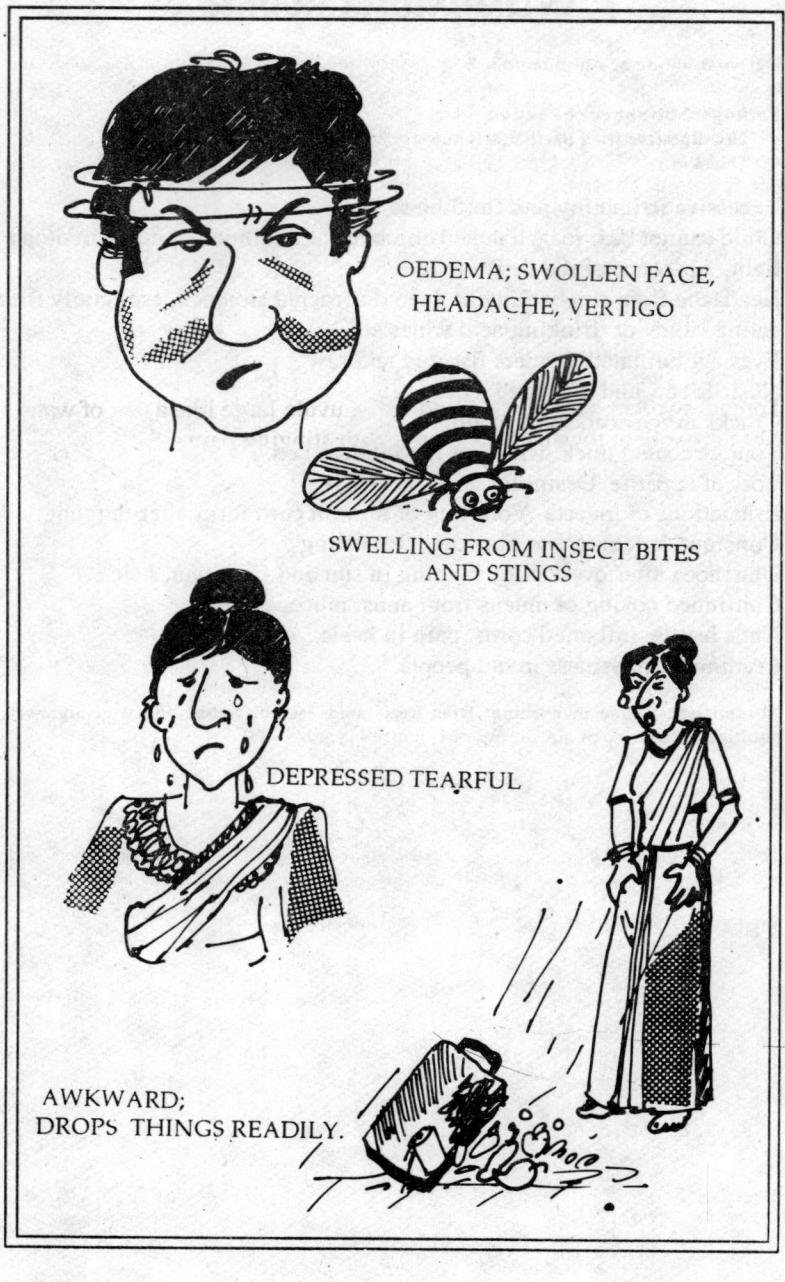

OEDEMA; SWOLLEN FACE, HEADACHE, VERTIGO

SWELLING FROM INSECT BITES AND STINGS

DEPRESSED TEARFUL

AWKWARD; DROPS THINGS READILY.

APIS MELLIFICA

Common name- Honey bee poison. N.O. Insecta.Tincture are made of whole bee and of dilutions of the poison with alcohol.

Pathogenetic sphere of action
- Oedema which may be generalised and may even spread into the mucosa.
- The serous membrane causing effusions.
- The renal parenchyma causing nephritis.

Awkwardness, drops things readily.

Great sadness, depression with constant weeping.

Lids swollen, oedematous, Photophobia.

Suppurative inflammation of eyes.

Face red, swollen, waxy, pale.

Tongue swollen, red, shining and puffy, uvula large like a bag of water.

Throat swollen, tonsils swollen, red with stinging pain.

Thirstlessness. Craving for milk.

Dropsy of abdomen, peritonitis.

Involuntary stools; anus seems wide open.

Urination painful and with burning, Urine high coloured and scanty, with blood, albumin and casts.

Oophritis, especially of right ovary.

Synovitis.

Swelling after bites, sore sensitive; stinging pain all over.

Erysipelas. Sudden puffing of whole body.

Very drowsy; sudden starting during sleep with screams.

Fever with afternoon chill with thirst.

Meningitis with "Cri-Encephlique".

Modalities: Worse heat, touch, pressure, late in afternoon, after sleeping, in closed and heated rooms, right side. Better in open air, uncovering and cold bathing.

Dosage : 3x for diuisetic effects, its sure. 30th and above otherwise.

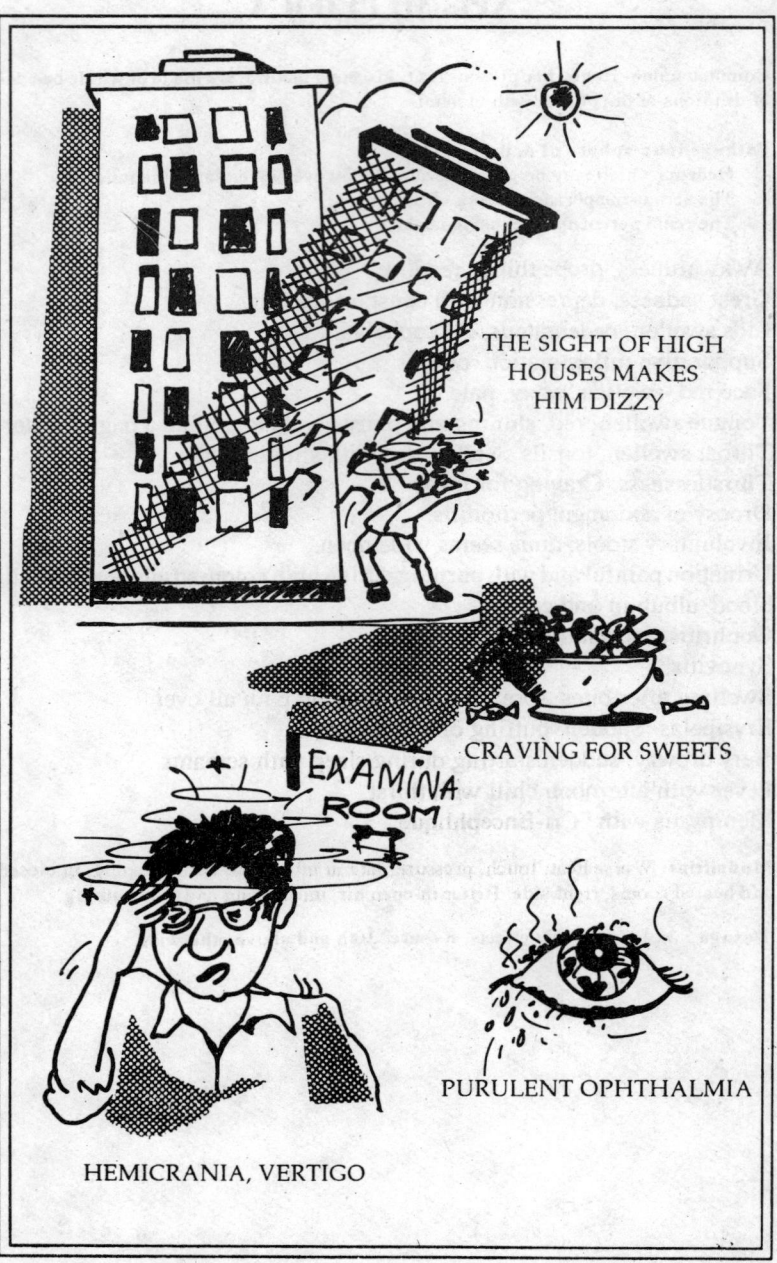

THE SIGHT OF HIGH
HOUSES MAKES
HIM DIZZY

CRAVING FOR SWEETS

EXAMINA
ROOM

PURULENT OPHTHALMIA

HEMICRANIA, VERTIGO

ARGENTUM NITRICUM

Nitrate of Silver. Lunar caustic AgNO$_3$ Trituration and solution.

Pathogenetic: sphere of action
- The nervous system causing asthenic, trembling and convulsions.
- The Mucous membranes causing inflammation. which leads to ulceration particularly in larynx, pharynx, stomach, intestines and genitals.

Fear of the unknown; fear of death. Nervousness.
Impulsive.
Time passes too slowly; wants to do things in a hurry.
Melancholic; sweats with anxiety; irrational thoughts.
The sights of high houses makes him dizzy.
Excitable; angers easily.
Memory weak. Mental exhaustion. Examination feat.
Headache with coldness and trembling.
Hemicrania from emotional disturbances.
Sense of expansion. headache better by tight bandaging
Vertigo on looking upwards.
Purulent ophthalmia, corneal ulcers, corneal opacities.
Weakened ciliary muscles. Accommodation difficult.
Face sunken - old man's look.
Sensation of splinter on throat - hawking thick mucus.
Great desire for sweets. Belching with most gastric complaints. Gastritis of drunkards.
Ulcer of stomach with radiating pain.
Diarrhoea, green like chopped spinach; fluids go right through him.
Chronic hoarseness; high notes cause cough.
Weariness and weakness of leg muscles, can't walk with eyes closed.
Rigidity of calves.
Post diptheritic paralysis.
Irregular blotches over skin.
Sleeplessness due to imaginary troubles.

Modalities: Worse Warmth. at night. from cold food, sweets, after eating, at menstrual period. from motions, left side.Better from eructation, fresh air, cold pressure.

Dosage : 30th for gastric complaints. Higher for nevous diseases.

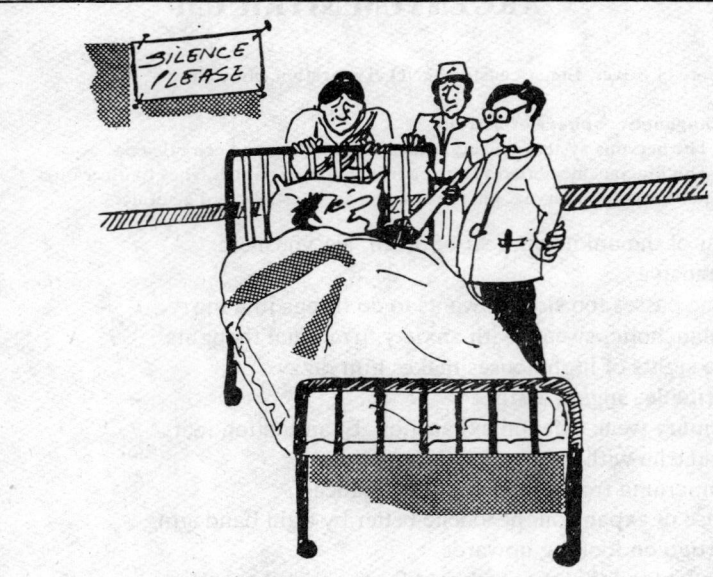

DELUSION; SAYS HE IS NOT SICK

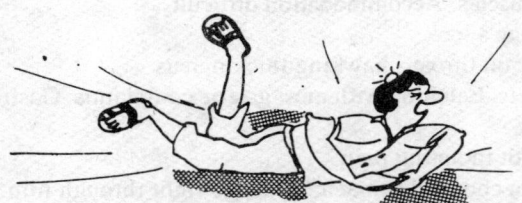

BRUISES, ECCHYMOSES & SPRAINS WITH
SORE LAME BRUISED FEELING

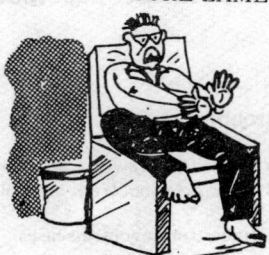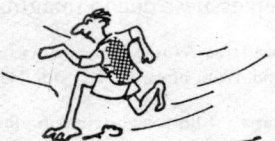

FEAR OF BEING TOUCHED OR APPROACHED

ARNICA MONTANA

Arnica montana. Common name leopard's bane. Fallkraut. N.O. compositae. Tincture of whole fresh plant. Tincture of root.

Pathogenetic: sphere of action
- Muscles and Cellular tissue producing soreness or aching sensations.
- The Capillaries. causing extra vasation of blood and ecchymoses.
- It causes an adynamic, febrile condition.

Pre-eminently a drug for bruises, sprains, strains and shock following injury, especially due to a fall.

Great fear of being touched. Gout.

Unconscious; when spoken to answers correctly but again goes to sleep.

Says there is nothing the matter with him.

Agoraphobia (fear of space). Indifference, head hot with cold body.

Cerebral concussion.

Retinal and sub conjunctival haemmorrhage.

Fetid breath from mouth, taste as from bad eggs.

Post - operative shock.

Vesical tenesmus, vesical injuries etc.

Bruised parts after labour.

Violent spasmodic cough with facial herpes, pleurŏdynia.

Angina pectoris, "Athlete's Heart" (dilatation of heart).

Skin - black and blue, crops of small recurring boils.

Bed sores - ecchymosis.

Typhoid and relapsing fevers; septicaemia.

Modalities: Worse least touch, motion, rest, wine, damp cold. Better, lying down, or with head low.

Dosage : 30th or 200th for injuries. Very high for thrombo-embolic phenomena. Its thrombolytic or fibrinolytic action im sure.

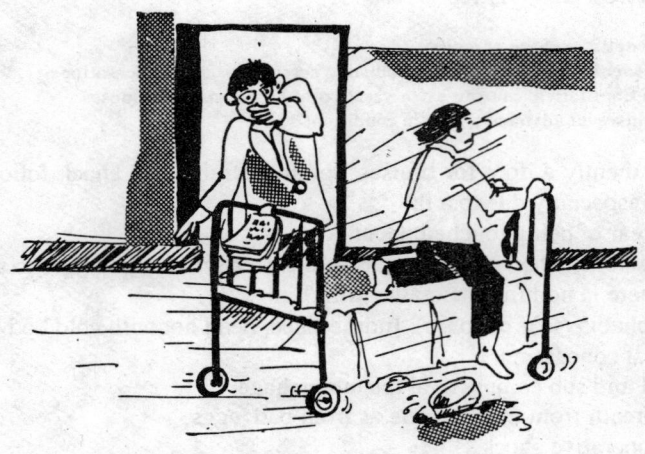

GREAT ANXIETY AND RESTLESSNESS
ESPECIALLY AFTER MIDNIGHT

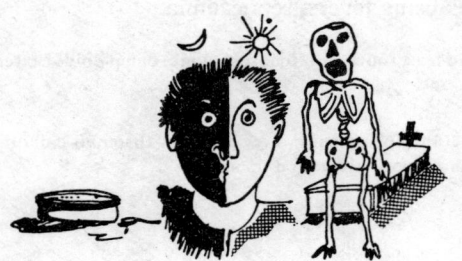

DREAD OF DEATH: SEES GHOSTS DAY & NIGHT
EXCESSIVE THIRST:
DRINKS MUCH,   BUT LITTLE AT A TIME

ARSENICUM ALBUM

The white oxide of Metallic Arsenic As_2O_3. Solution and trituration.

Pathogenetic: Sphere of action
- The mucosa causing inflammation with tendency to necrotic ulceration.
- The vital organs causing damage to their parenchyma.
- The nervous system causing convulsions and coma and progressive paraly sis with cramps.
- The skin causing dryness, induration, and squamous eruptions.
- The circulatory system.
- There is weakening of vital functions causing weight loss, ashtenia, anaemia.

Marked physical and mental restlessness, worse after midnight.
Great anxiety, changes places continually.
Fear of death. Suicidal mania.
Sensitive to disorder and confusion.
Burning pain in head, relieved by cold.
Thin, watery, excoriating coryza.
Ulceration of mouth with blue colour with fetid breath.
Vomiting, if any thing cold drink taken.
Thirst marked; drinks often but little.
Can't bear the sight and smell of food.
Burning pain in stomach.
Ill effects of vegetable diet, melons etc.
Liver and spleen enlarged and tender.
Diarrhoea with much prostration, worse during night and after eating or drinking.
Bright's disease.
Asthma, alternating with eczema; worse after mid night.
Pulse more rapid in morning.
Itching and burning, better warm application.
Fever - intermittent with marked exhaustiion.
Great heat about 3 A.M.

Modalities: Worse wet weather, after midnight from cold, cold drinks, food, seashore right side. Better from heat, from head elevated, warm drinks.

Dosage : 30th few doses. Higher infrequent if required.

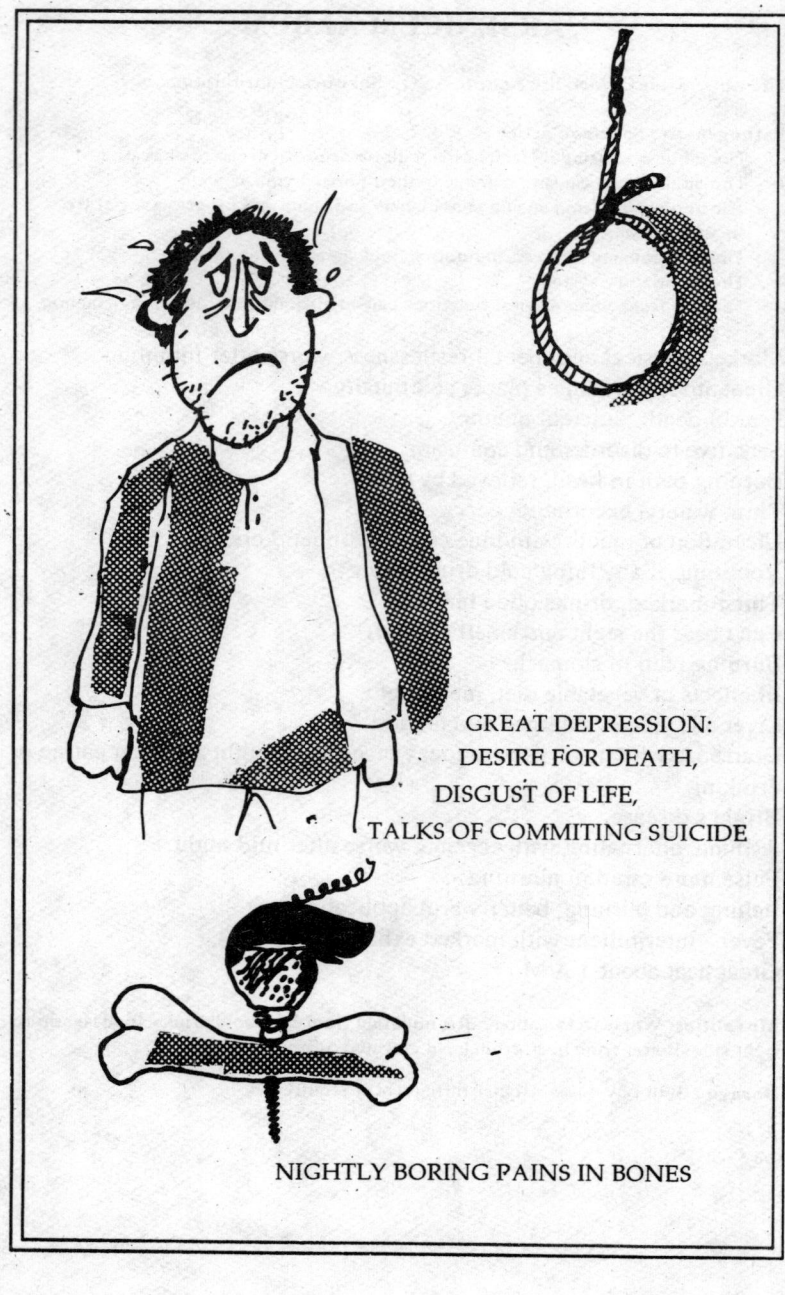

GREAT DEPRESSION:
DESIRE FOR DEATH,
DISGUST OF LIFE,
TALKS OF COMMITING SUICIDE

NIGHTLY BORING PAINS IN BONES

AURUM METALLICUM

Aurum foliatum (Metallic gold) Au. (A.W.1968). Trituation.

Patogenetic sphere of action
- The nervous system causing depression.
- The Circulation causing a hypertensive tendency and Cardiomegaly.
- The short bones causing exostoses and cavities.
- The lymphatic and glandular tissues causing hypertrophy and induration.

Profound despondency. Feeling of self condemnation.
Disgust for life. Always talks of committing suicide.
Oversensitiveness; to noise excitement.
Violent pain in head, worse at night.
Extreme photophobia; upper half of objects invisible.
Interstitial keratitis, sticking pain in eyes.
Profuse, obstinate, fetid otorrhoea.
Nose - ulcerated, painful, putrid discharge from nose.
Angina pectoris, Hypertension and violent palpitation, arteriosclerotic valvular diseases.
Pulse, rapid and irregular.
Dyspnoea at night.
Chronic induration of testicles.
Destruction of bones. Pain bones wakes the patient from sleep. Deep boring pains in bones.
Sleeplessness.

Modalities: Worse in Cold weather, when getting cold, in winters sunset to sunrise.

Dosage : 200th infrequent doses.

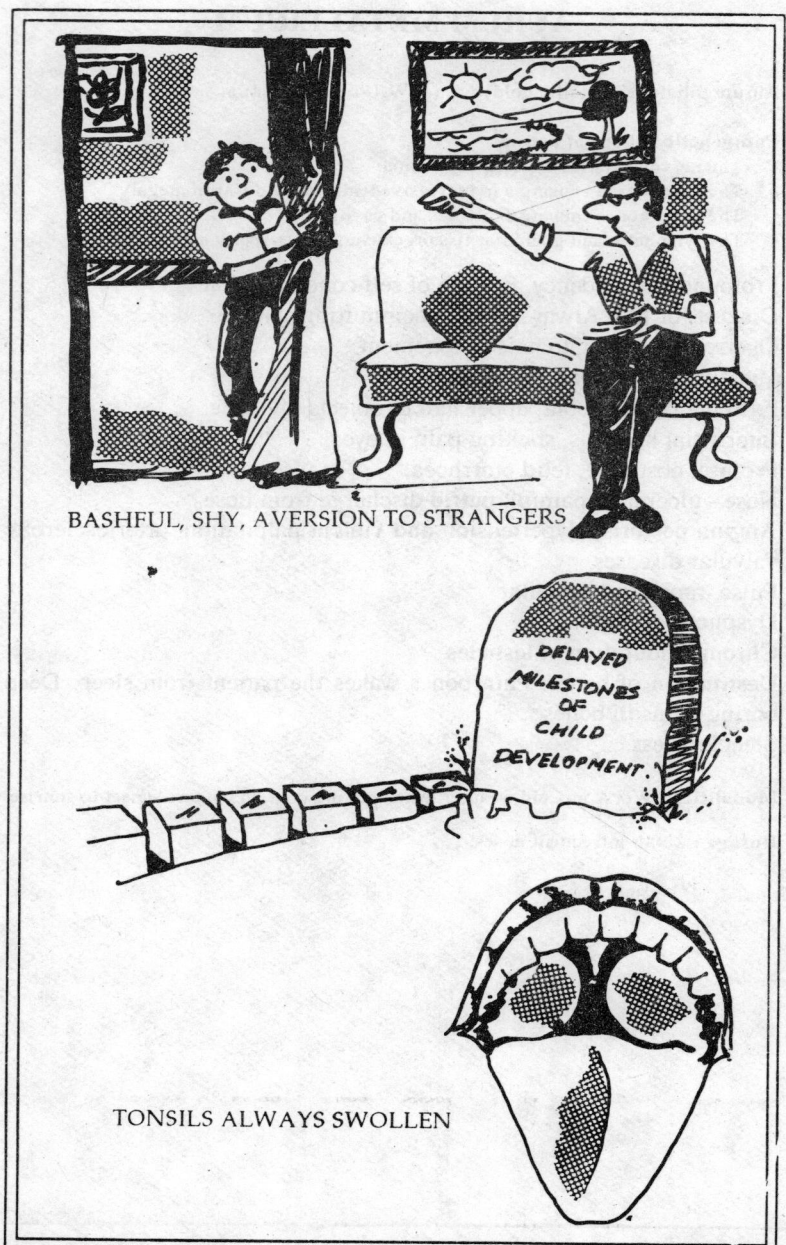

BASHFUL, SHY, AVERSION TO STRANGERS

DELAYED
MILESTONES
OF
CHILD
DEVELOPMENT

TONSILS ALWAYS SWOLLEN

BARYTA CARBONICA

Carbonate of Barium $BaCO_3$, with which are included symptoms of Baryta acetica - Barium acetate $Ba(C_2H_3O_2)_2$. Trituration of carbonate, solution of acetate is used.

Pathogenetic: sphere of action
- Patients's general development causing physical and intellectual backward ness.
- The Circulatory system causing degenerative action upon the arterial walls.
- The lymphatic system causing hypertrophy of tonsils, sclerosis of prostrate gland.

Specially indicated in the extremes of life i.e. in infancy and old age.
Children who do not grow and develop properly.
All the milestones of development are delayed.
Children, backward mentally as well as physically.
Mentally weak, shy and averse to strangers.
Childish behaviour.
Lymphatic glands around ears swollen and tender.
Crackling noises in ear.
Tongue thick, Swollen, protruded with dribbling of saliva.
Tonsils always enlarged and swollen.
Very susceptible to take cold. Quinsy.
Suppurative tonsillitis from every cold with sticking pain, worse empty swallowing.
Spasms of oesophagus.
Abdomen distended, hard and tense.
Enlarged mesentric glands.
Chronic cervical lymphadenitis.
Fetid foot sweats.

Modalities: Worse, while thinking of symptoms, from washing, lying on painful side.Better, walking in open air.

Dosage : 200th twice daily. Prolonged administration is required owing to recurrent tendecy to catch infection (initially). 1M or higher to eradiccate tendecy to septic throat complaints.

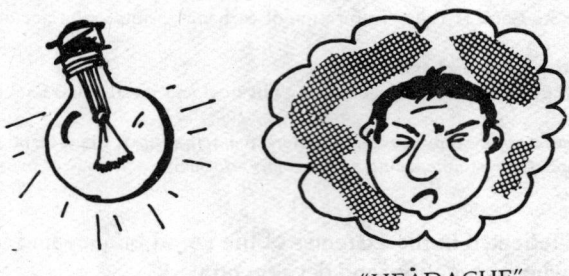

"HEADACHE"

LEAST NOISE, LIGHT ANNOYING

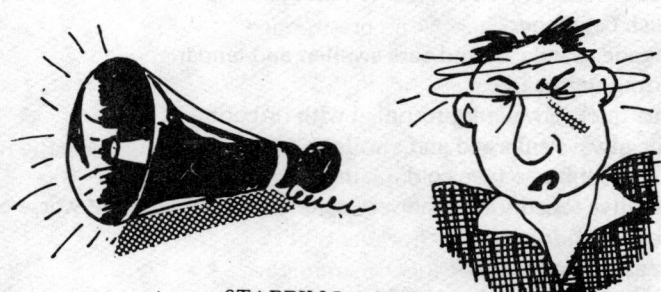

STABBING & THROBBING HEADACHE

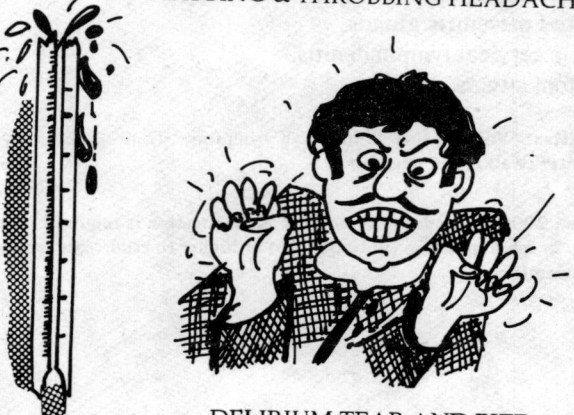

DELIRIUM TEAR AND BITE

GREAT, SUDDEN HEAT WITH BURNING STEAMING HEAT

BELLADONNA

Commonly called Atropa Belladonna Common name – Deadly night shade.N.O. solanaceae. Tincture of whole plant when beginning to flower.

Pathogenetic sphere of action
- The mucous membrane causing dryness.
- The circulatory system causing local or general vascular congestion.
- The nervous system causing violent angry delirium with hallucinations.

Heat, redness, excited mental state, sudden development and hyperaesthesia of all senses.

Furious; Delirium, with tendency to bite and strike, desire to escape. Visual hallucinations.

Violent throbbing headache, especially in forehead; with throbbing carotids; worse light, noise, jar, lying down etc., better by pressure.

Face flushed and hot.

Pupils dilated, red, staring and protruding.

Otitis media, pain, violent, makes the patient mad.

Child cries out while sleeping.

Grinding of teeth while sleeping.

Throat inflamed, congested. Tonsils enlarged, inflamed, especilly right sided, with great difficulty in swallowing.

Great thirst for cold water, but dread of drinking.

Short dry, tickling cough; worse at night.

High feverish states. Burning, steaming heat.

Epileptic convulsion in children and infants.

"Air sickness", often works as preventive for avaitors.

Modalities: Worse touch, jar, noise, draught, afternoon, lying down. Better semi erect.

Dosage : 3x in acute inflammation, repeatedly. 200th or higher in psychiatric ailments infrequently.

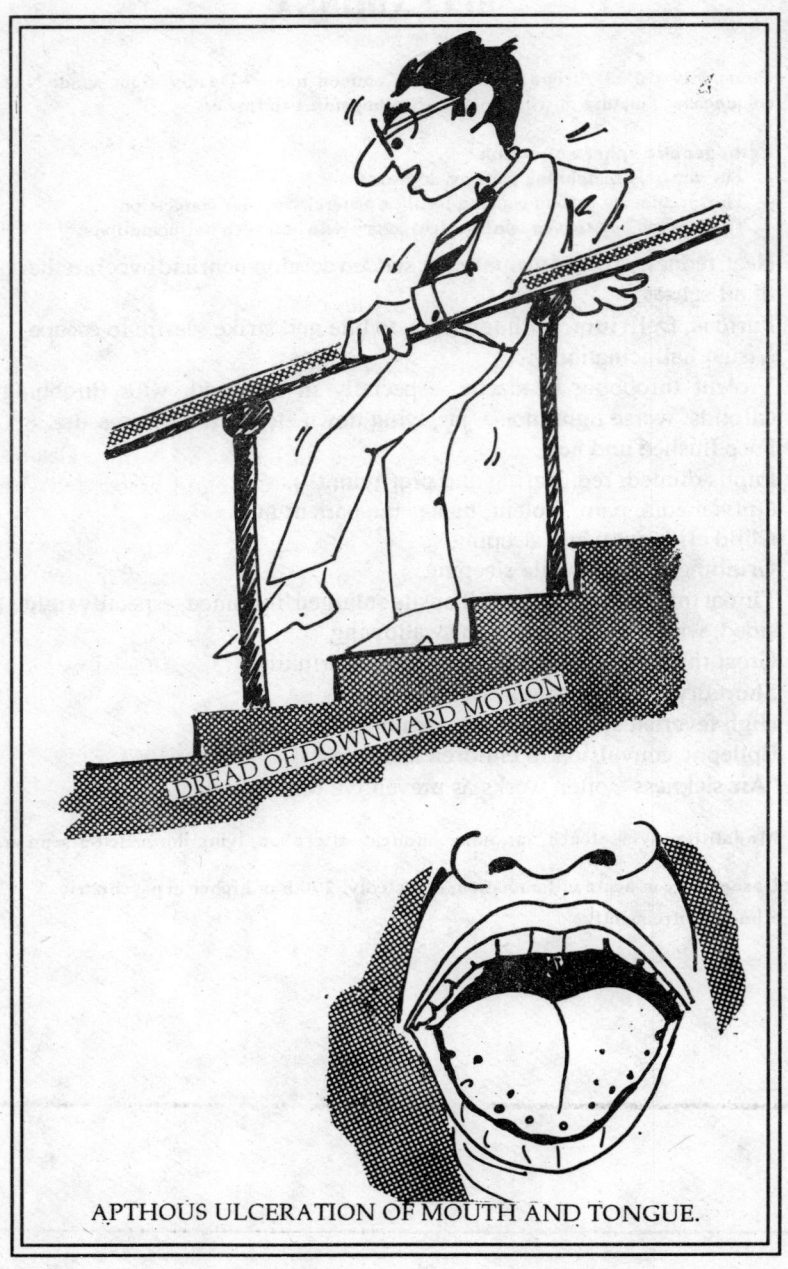

DREAD OF DOWNWARD MOTION

APTHOUS ULCERATION OF MOUTH AND TONGUE.

BORAX

Natrum biboracicum. It is prepared by Trituration and solution.

Pathogenetic: sphere of action
- The Mucosa particularly of the mouth causing aphtous ulcers.
- The skin causing vesicular eruptions.
- The Nervous system causing hypersensitivity to sudden loud noises, fear of down ward motion, falling.

Dread of downward motion in nearly all complaints.
Apthous ulceration of mucous membranes.
Extreme anxiety, especially from motion having downward direction e.g. coming down in lift, rocking, laid down, coming down stairs etc.
Sensitive to sudden noises. even slightest.
Apthae; mouth hot, tender, ulcers bleed on touch and eating. Gastrointestinal irritation, loose, pappy, offensive stool in child, associated with apthae.
Galactorrhoea; helps in drying up milk when weaning. Sterility; Membranous dysmenorrhoea; Menses too soon, profuse, with griping, nausea and pain in stomach. Leucorrhoea like white of an egg; as if warm water flowing.
Psoriasis. Eczema. Itching on back of finger joints. Unhealthy skin. Allergic dermatitis on finger and hands.

Modalities: Worse from; downward motion, noise, smoking, warm weather, after menses, Better pressure, evening, cold weather.

Dosage : 30th or 200th few doses.

34

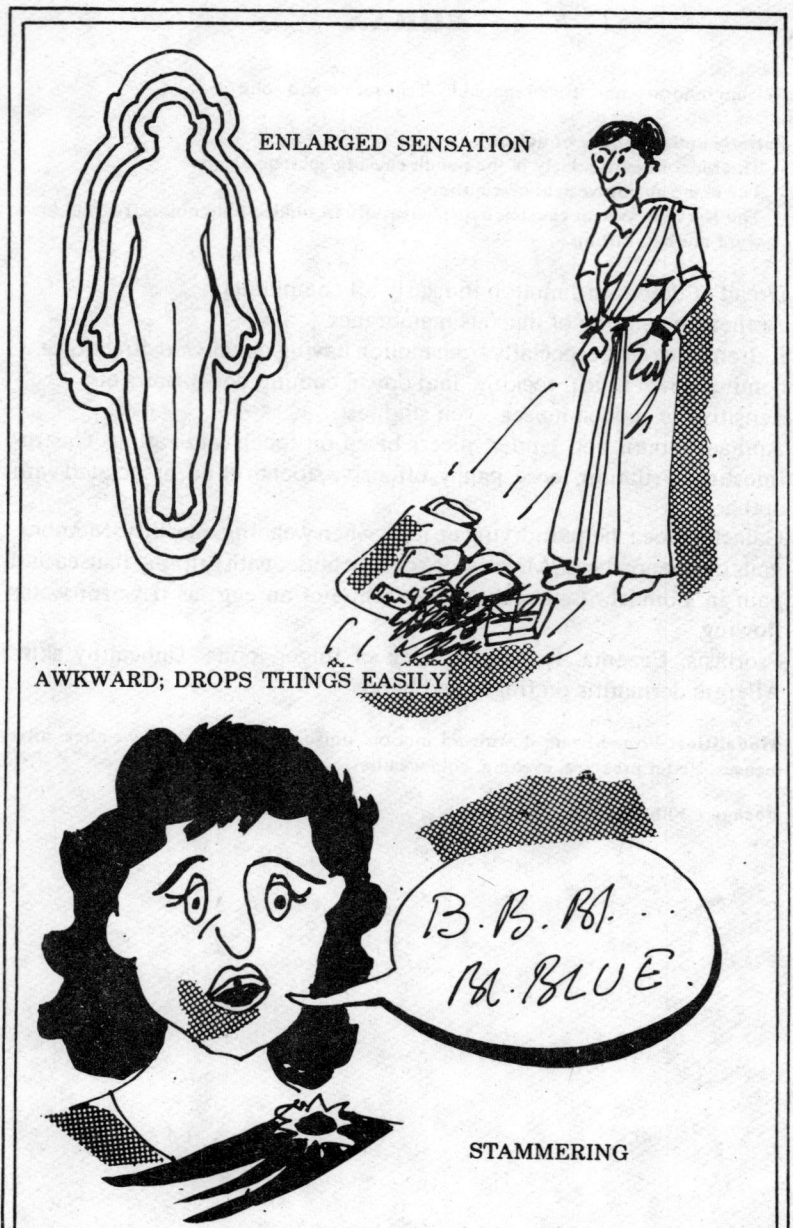

BOVISTA

Lycoperdon Bovista.Warted puff ball N.O. Fungi.Trituration

Pathogenetic sphere of action
- Female genital system causing functional intermenstrual bleeding.
- Digestive system.

It is suited to stammering children, old maids with palpitationand tettery patients.
Sensation as if everything is enlarged.
Awkward, everything falls from hands.
Sensation as if head were enlarging especially of occiput.
Discharge from nose is stringy, tough.
Acne worse in summer due to use of cosmetics
Diarrhoea before and during menses.
Menses too early and profuse worse at night.
Cannot bear tight clothing around waist
Traces of memses between mensturation
Colic with red urine relieved by eating.
Sweat in axilla smelling like onions.
Tip of coccyx itches intolerably.
Urticaria on excitement with rheumatic lameness, palpitation and diarrhoea.

Modalities: Worse in summer.

Dosage : 30th or 200th 3 times a day.

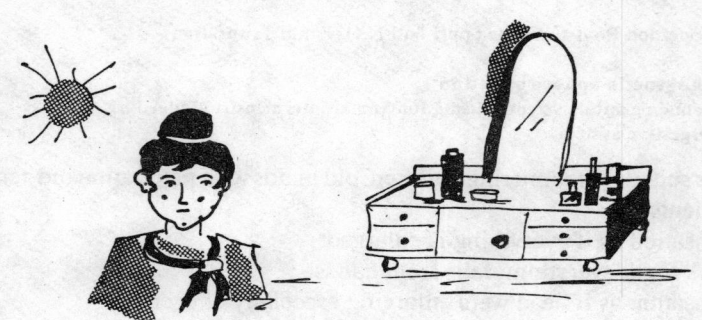

ACNE, WORSE - SUMMER, USE OF COSMETICS

LEFT SIDED MUMPS

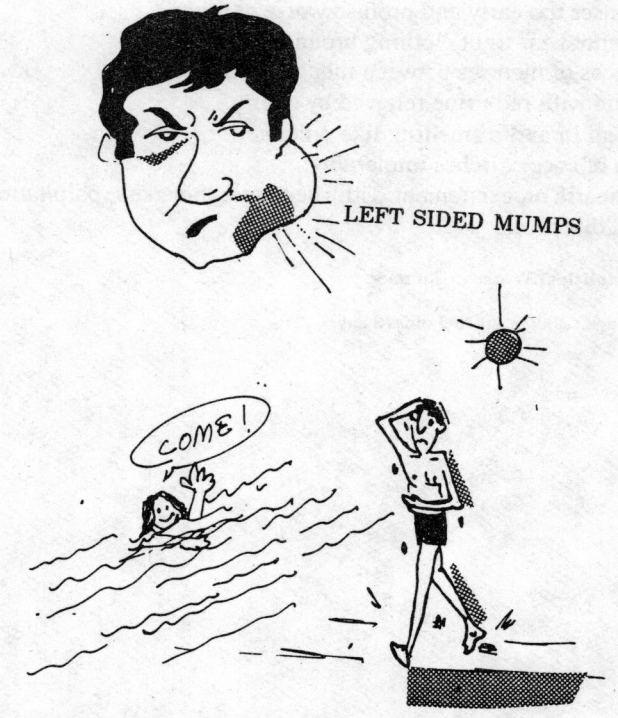

BETTER AT SEA; WORSE AT SEASHORE (ASTHMA)

BROMIUM

Bromine Br (A.W.79.9) solutionin distilled water.

Pathogenetic Sphere of action
- The Mucosa causing irriation ranging from dry excoriating inflammation to formation of false membranes.
- The lymphatic system causing swelling, induration and indolence.
- Nervous system causing sadness and depression.

It affects the blond type.

There is tendency to infiltrate glands, become hard but seldom suppurate.

There is tickling, smarting in nose as from cobwebs.

Dry Cough with hoarseness and burning pain behind sternum.

Spasmodic cough with ratting of mucus in the larynx, suffocative.

Hoarseness.

There is cold sensation when inspiring

Laryngeal diptheria, membrane begins in larynx and spreads upward.

Asthma - difficulty in getting air into lung.

Glands story hard especially on lower jaw and throat.

Modalities: Worse from evening, until midnight, when sitting in warm room, warm damp weather, at rest and lying on left side. Better from any motion, exercise, at sea.

Dosage : 30th 3-4 times a day.

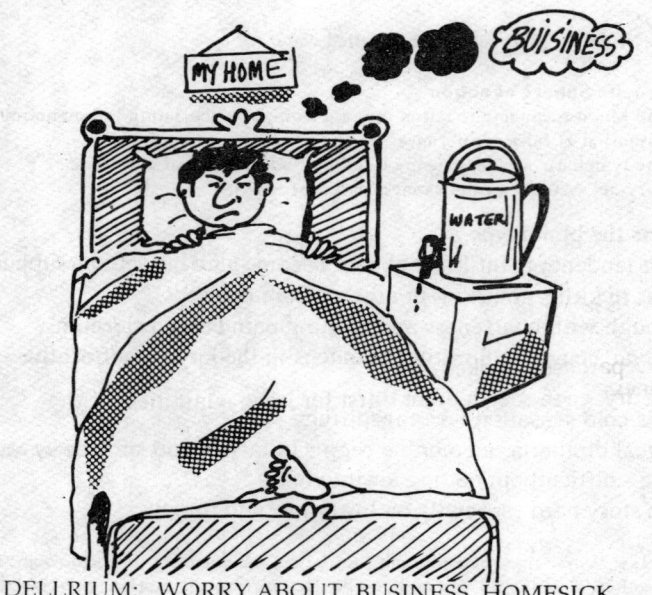

DELLRIUM: WORRY ABOUT BUSINESS, HOMESICK,
GREAT THIRST

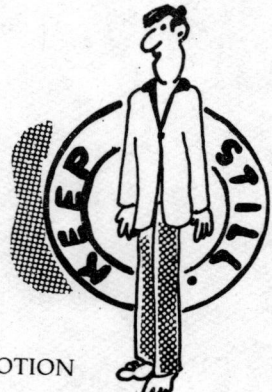

PAINS WORSE BY SLIGHTEST MOTION

BRYONIA ALBA

Common name white Bryony. N.O. Cucurbitaceae. Tincture of root procured before flowering.

Pathogenetic sphere of action
- The mucosa - causing dryness particularly in respiratory and digestive tract with intensive thirst.
- The serous membrane causing exudation.

Great irritability. Always worried about his business.

Delusions; wants to go home.

Vertigo, in morning on rising.

Bursting, splitting Headache esp. in morning.

Lips dry, parched, cracked.

Tongue dry, coated with great thirst for large quantities of water.

Nausea and vomiting in morning.

Pressure in stomach after eating, stomach becomes sensitive to touch with vomiting of bile.

Liver enlarged and painful. Stitching pain worse coughing, breathing etc.

Constipation - stool hard, dry as if burnt.

Dry cough at night, must sit up and hold the chest.

Stitching pain in chest.

Dry pleurisy.

Stiffness in small of back.

Joints red, swollen, effusion in joints.

All complaints are worse by least movement.

Modalities: Worse: warmth, any motion, morning, eating, hot weather, exertion, touch, cannot sit gets faint and sick. Better lying on painful side, pressure, rest, cold things.

Dosage : 6 for actue complaints. 10M for arthritic complaints esp. Osteoarthritis.

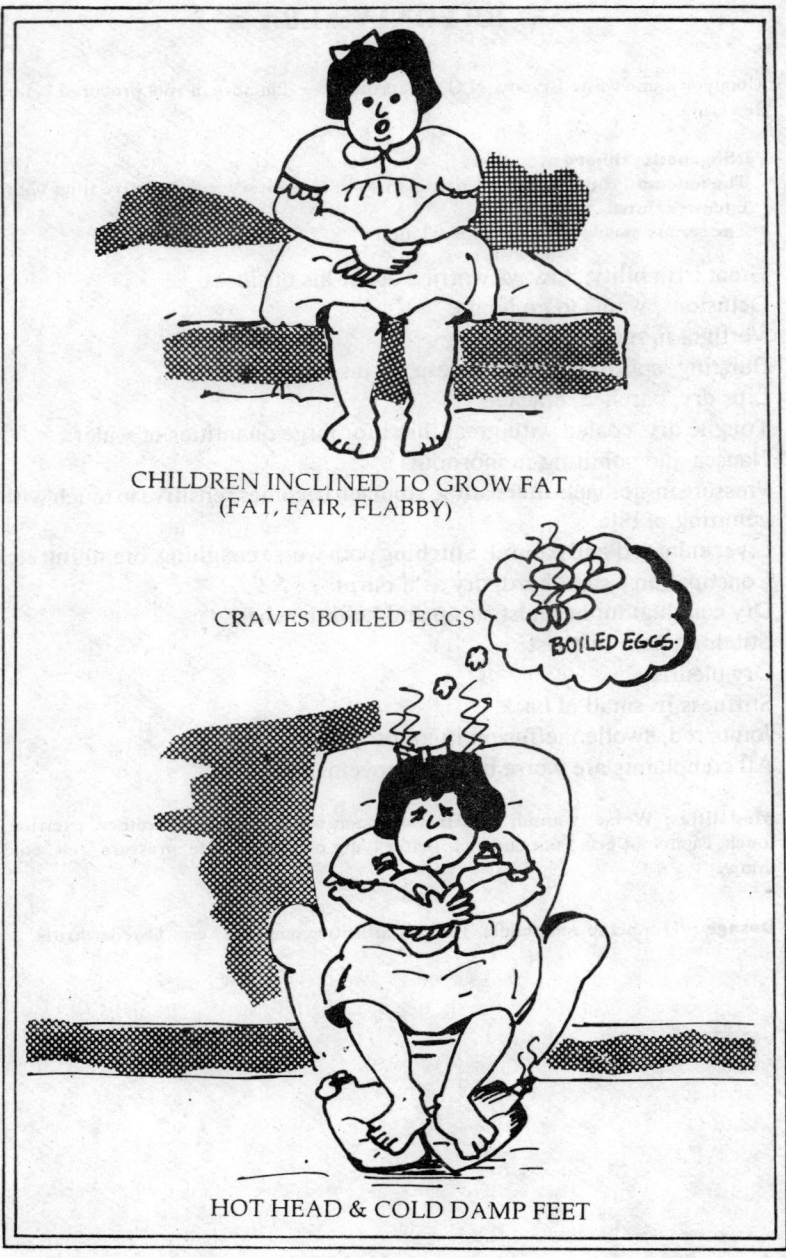

CHILDREN INCLINED TO GROW FAT
(FAT, FAIR, FLABBY)

CRAVES BOILED EGGS

BOILED EGGS.

HOT HEAD & COLD DAMP FEET

CALCAREA CARBONICA

Impure Calcium Carbonate $CaCO_3$. It includes symptoms of calcarea acetica and Calcarea ostrearum, a trituration of middle layer of oyster shells.

Pathgenetic: sphere of action
- Bone tissue producing deformation and exostoses.
- The lymphoid tissue in general and especially lymph nodes in neck causing hypertrophy with a tendency towards inflammation and suppuration.
- The circulatory system causing anaemia and local congestive phenomenon, feet cold and heat hot, congestion of chest.
- Polyps of nose, vagina, bladder etc.

Fat, fair, flabby, sweating and chilly child.
Delayed dentition, rickets.
Low spirited, Melacholic, sad and worried about future.
"Fears that something sad or terrible will happen."
Child cross and fretful, easily frightened.
Aversion to work -physical as well as mental.
Profuse sweat on head upon slightest exertion, wets the pillow.
Headche from mental exertion. Sensation of weight and ice, on top of head. Delayed closure of fontanalles.
Vertigo from mental exertion.
Thick scabs on the head, with yellow and offensive discharge from eruptions.
Disturbance of accomodation. Dim vision.
Headache from eye strain and mental exertion.
Ear troubles with muco-purulent otorrhoea and enlarged glands around ears. Cracking noises in ear.
Nasal polypi; profuse coryza from slightest cold.
Face pale, and sickly. All cervical lymph glands are enlarged. Goitre.
Chronic sore taste in mouth.
Craving for indigestible things-chalk, coal etc. and for eggs, salt and sweets. Aversion for fat. Milk disagrees.
Sour vomiting and eructations.
Abdomen distended with liver enlarged and painful.
Umbilical hernia, gall bladder colic and renal colic.
Constipation; children's diarrhoea. Stools first hard then pasty and then liquid, white clay coloured.
Menses too early, too short, too profuse and long lasting with milky leucorrhoea and damp icy cold feet. Galactorrhoea.
Rheumatoid Arthritis; Cold extremities. Soles of feet raw.
Sleep greatly disturbed.

Modalities: Worse form exertion, mental or physical, ascending, cold in every form, water, washing, moist air, wet weather, during full moon, standing. Better in dry climate and weather, lying on painful side.

Dosage : 200th few doses or higher. Deep remedy. Wait for its action.

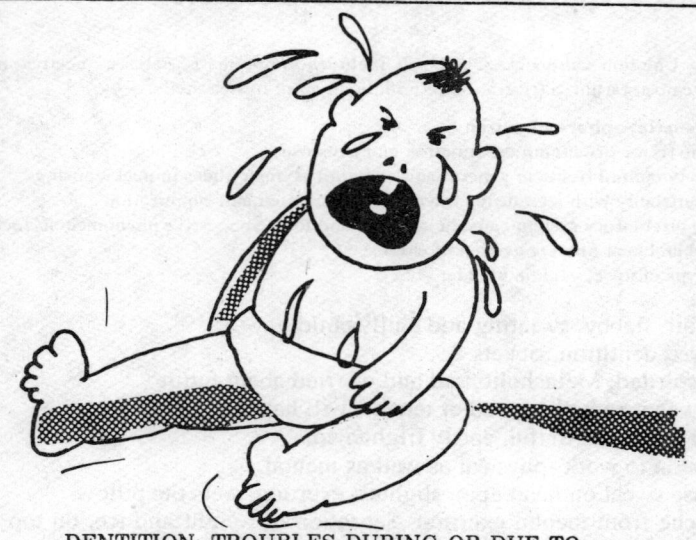

DENTITION; TROUBLES DURING OR DUE TO

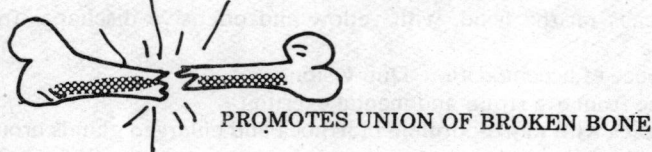

PROMOTES UNION OF BROKEN BONE

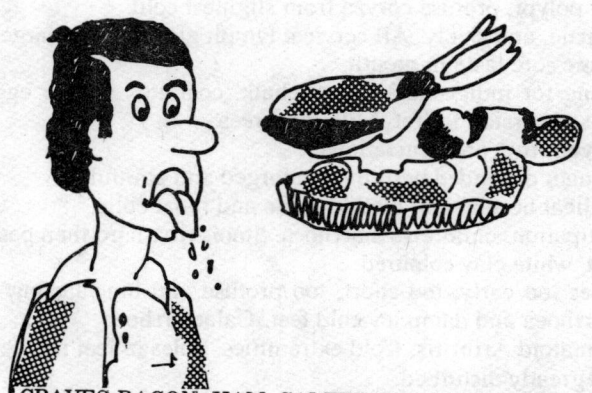

CRAVES BACON, HAM, SALTED OR SMOKED MEAT

CALCAREA PHOSPHORICA

Phosphate of lime Ca$_3$ 2PO$_4$. A mixture of the basic and others phosphates of lime made by dropping dilute phosphoric acid into lime water,Trituration.

Pathogenetic sphere of action
- The bony tissues causing growth disorders or disorders attributed to adolescence teething, slow healing fractures, dystrophy.
- The blood and lymph nodes.
- The nutrition - causing weight loss, rickets etc.

Anaemic children who are peevish, flabby have cold extremities and feeble digestion.

Numbness and crawling sensation.

Headache worse near the region of sutures, from change of weather.

Adenoid growths.

Craving for bacon, ham, salted or smoked meat.

Much flatulence.

At every attempt to eat, colicky pain in abdomen.

Stools are greenish, slimy, hot, sputtering undigested with foetid flatus.

Stiffness and pain with numb and cold feeling in extremities.

Modalities: Worse exposure to damp, cold weather, melting Snow. Better in summer, warm, dry atmosphere

Dosage : 3x or 6x, 2 to 3 times daily.

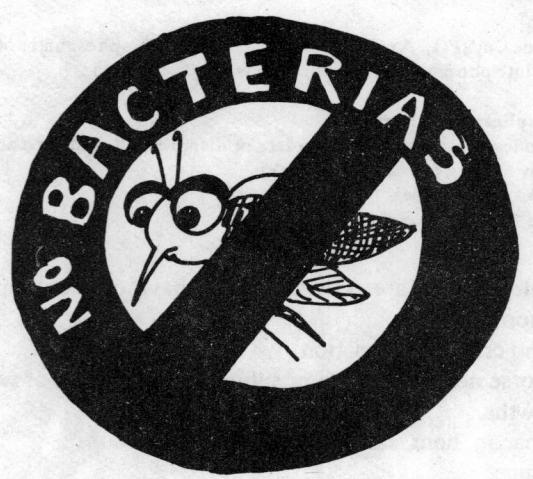

BACTERIOSTATIC   A MOST VALUABLE HEALING AGENT

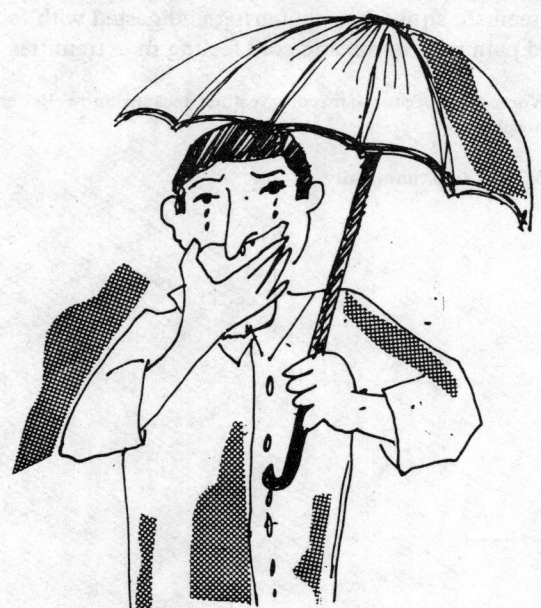

CATCHES COLD EASILY ESPECIALLY IN DAMP WEATHER

CALENDULA OFFICINALIS

Common name Marigold. N.O. compositae.Tincture of leaves and flowers.

Pathogenetic sphere of action
- Externally as an antiseptic and cicatrizing agent.
- Internally it has antiseptic action upon lacerated wounds and infected ulcers.

Bacteriostatic properties; do not allow any bacterial growth on wound; hence no pus formation; no scar.

Minimize scarring of skin following injury. Promotes healthy granulation and rapid healing.

For burns, sores, fissures, ulcers, abrasions, open wounds, lacerated scalp wound. Stops haemorrhoids

Great disposition to take cold, especially in damp climate.

Hears best on a train, and distant sounds.

Chronic endocervictis,cervical erosion.

Modalities: Worse in damp, heavy, cloudy weather.

Dosage : 30th internally. Lotion (1:9) in distilled water for local applications.

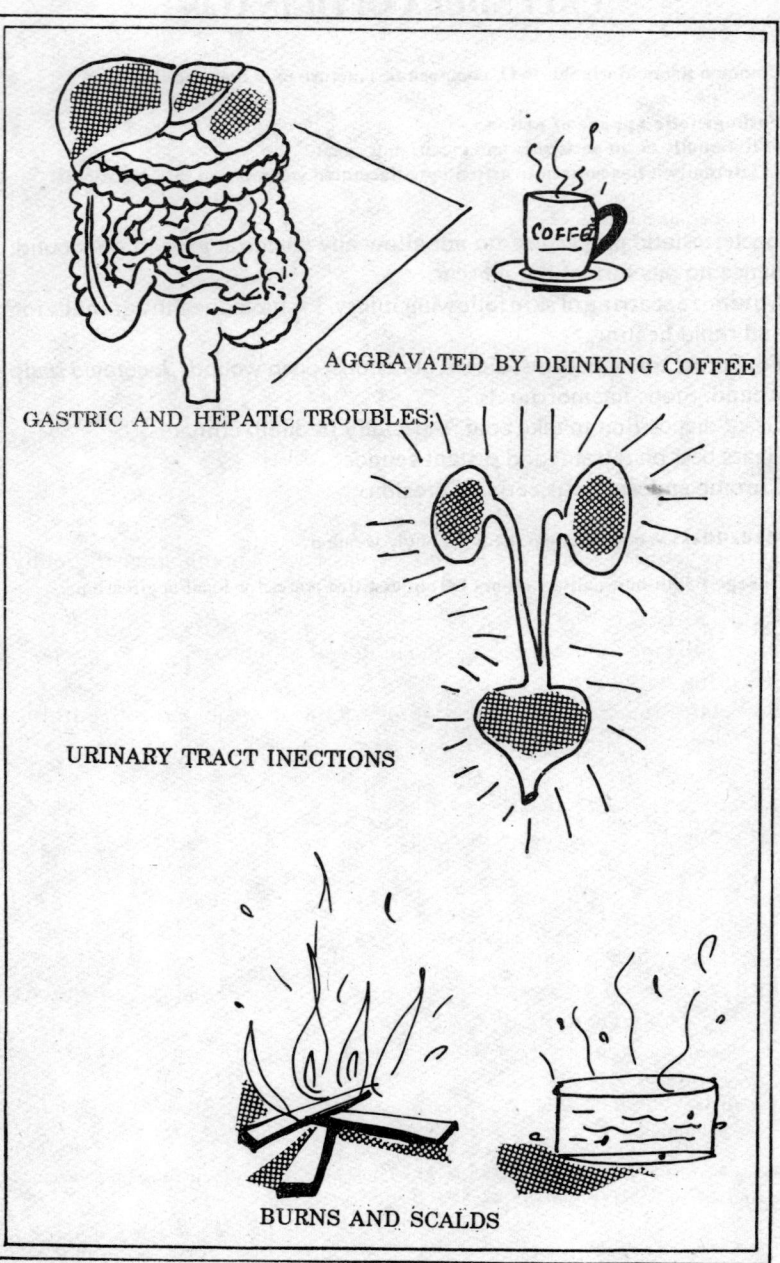

GASTRIC AND HEPATIC TROUBLES; AGGRAVATED BY DRINKING COFFEE

URINARY TRACT INECTIONS

BURNS AND SCALDS

CANTHARIS

Cantharis vesicator. Spanish fly N.O. Insecta, Coleoptera. Tincture or trituration of living insects.

Pathogenetic sphere of action
- The genito urinary tract causing acute inflammatory condition with intense burning and vesiculation which may reach the point of gangrene.
- The serous membranes causing exudations.
- The skin causing extremely burning vesiculo-bullous eruptions.

Raw burning pains.

Intolerable, constant urging to urinate.

Gastric, hepatic, abdominal complaints are aggravated by drinking coffee.

Acute mania, generally of sexual type, amorous frenzy, fiery, sexual desire.

Sudden loss of conciousness with red face.

There is fiery, sparkling, staring look in eyes.

Burning in mouth, pharynx and throat, vesicles in mouth, great difficulty in swallowing liquids, very tenacious mucus.

Tendency to syncope.

Short, hacking cough blood streaked tenacious mucus.

Shivering with burning.

Dysentery, mucous stools like scrapings of intestines, blood with burning, and tenesmus and shuddering after stool.

Intolerable urging and tenesmus in urine.

Urine scalds him and is passed drop by drop, constant desire to urinate Strong desire; painful erections.

Nymphomania.

Pleurisy with exudation.

Pericarditis with effusion.

Vesicular eruptions with burning and Itching.

Burns, Scalds with rawness and smarting relieved by cold applications followed by undue inflammation.

Erysipelas, vesicular type with great restlessness.

Modalities: Worse form touch, or approach, urinating, drinking cold water or coffee. Better rubbing.

Dosage : 6th to 13th potency. Bears repeated doses well. Locally, in burns and eczema, IX and 2x, in water, or as cerate.

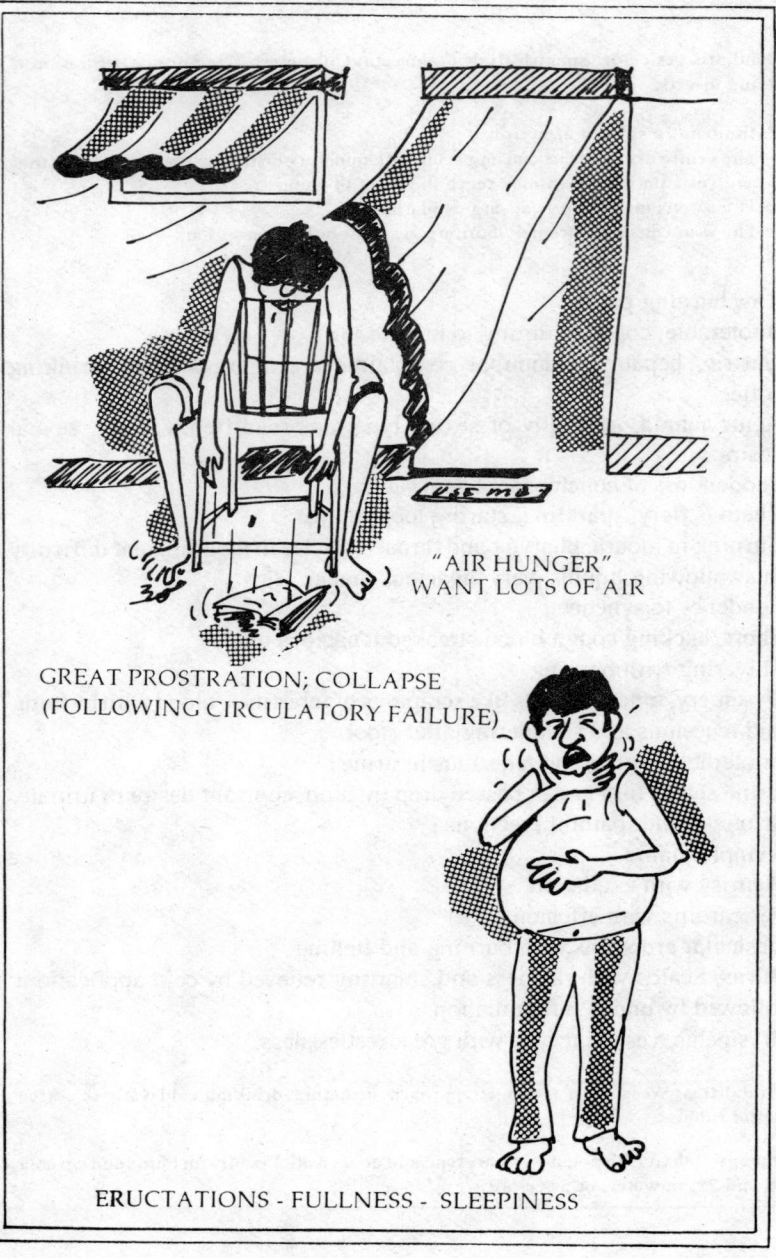

"AIR HUNGER"
WANT LOTS OF AIR

GREAT PROSTRATION; COLLAPSE
(FOLLOWING CIRCULATORY FAILURE)

ERUCTATIONS - FULLNESS - SLEEPINESS

CARBO VEGETABILIS

Commonly called vegetable charcoal. It is prepared by trituration.

Pathogenetic sphere of action
- The digestive tract causing flatulence with an unpleasant smell.
- The circulatory system causing slowness with venous stagnation, hypoxemia and cyanosis of extremities.
- Passive haemorrhage of black colour.
- The nervous system causing exhaustion, general weakness, prostration and a tendency to collapse and faint.

Lowered vital powers from loss of vital fluids and chronic diseases. Patients who have never recovered from the effects of some previous disease.

Headache mostly occipital from any exertion.

Hair fall out by the handful.

Face pale, cynotic, hippocratic, cold with cold sweat.

Epistaxis, with pale, anaemic face.

Great distention of upper part of abdomen. Slow digestion, food putrifies, eructations with fullness and heaviness.

Aversion to fat, milk, meat etc.

Flatulent colic.

Acrid and corrosive oozing of mucus from anus.

Diarrhoea very exhausting.

Bronchial asthma whooping cough, hoarsenes, worse evening.

Breath cold. Must be fanned constantly.

Skin blue, ecchymosed with cold sweat.

Senile gangrene. Varicose ulcers, carbuncles.

Shock and collapse with cold breath, cold tongue, cold face - looks like a "cadaver" - with all this there is great burning internally.

Wants a lot of air, wants to be fanned constantly.

Modalities: Worse in evening, night and open air, cold, fat food, butter, coffee, milk, warm damp weather, wine. Better from eructation, from fanning, cold.

Dosage : 30th few doses daily.

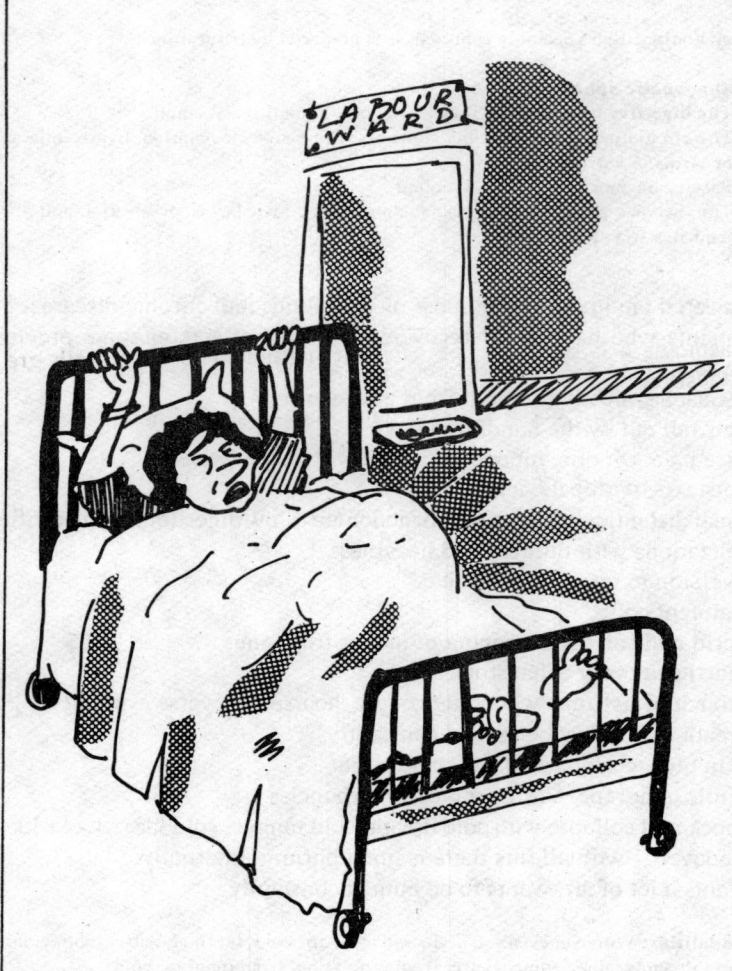

DURING LABOUR: PAINS ARE DEFICIENT AND
THE PATIENT IS EXHAUSTED AND IRRITABLE.

CAULOPHYLLUM

Caulophyllum thalictroides. Blue Cohosh, Squaw Root N.O. Berberidacea. Tincture or trituration of root.

Pathogenetic sphere of action

- The female genital system causing functional dysmenorrhoea with spasmodic pains of cervico-isthmic origin in women having light periods and who suffer on first day of mensturation

  It causes rheumatic pains in small articulartions, these are intermittent, paroxysmal and erratic. Changing place every 5 minutes.

Hysterical, fretful woman of hysterical and rheumatic consitution. Extraordinary rigidity of OS.

Spasmodic and severe labor pains but inefficient to expel, with great exhaustion.

Habitual abortion due to incompetent OS or weak uterine muscles.

Great atony of uterus. Severe after pains.

Protracted lochial discharge.

Dysmenorrhoea. Leucorrhoea.

Discoloration of skin in woman having uterine disorders.

Severe pain in small joints, especially carpal and metacarpal joints.

Stiffness and aching in wrist.

Modalities : Worse fear, anxiety. Better : passing discharges, warmth.

Dosage : 30th in later month of pregnancy, prepares for natural labor.

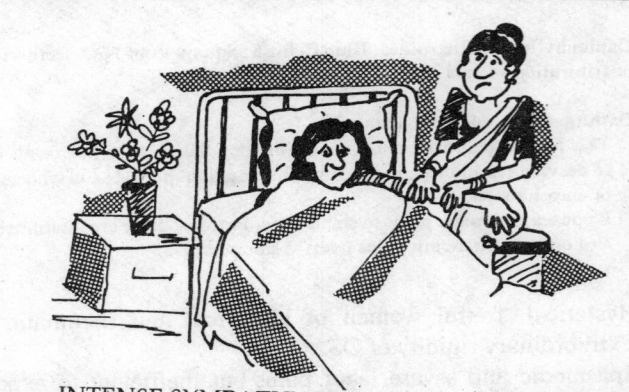

INTENSE SYMPATHY FOR OTHER'S SUFFERINGS

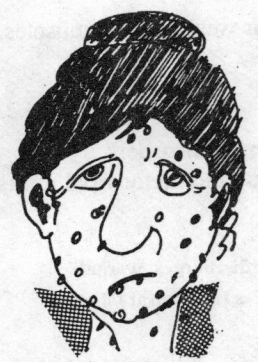

MELANCHOLIC; WARTS
AND ACNE ON FACE

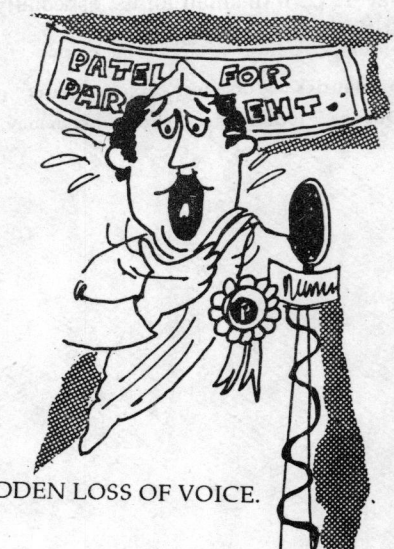

SUDDEN LOSS OF VOICE.

CAUSTICUM

Tinctura acris sine kali. Potassium hydrate. It is prepared by distilling a mixture of slaked lime and a solution of potassium sulphate. Tincture with spirit.

Pathogenetic sphere of action
- Cerebrum, motor area.
- Severe general weakness.
- Paralysis of isolated areas particularly of the face, larynx and sphincters.
- There is extensive paralysis coming on slowly and progressively.
- It has right sided progressive, hemiparesis and hemiplegia.

Intense sympathy for other's ailments.
Always anticipating some dreadful event.
Anxiety before falling asleep. Great sadness and weeping.
Mental and other complaints from long lasting grief and sorrow.
Tired, old, broken people, from prolonged struggle in business etc.
Facial paralysis of right side.
Paralysis of eye muscles, ptosis, diplopia. dim vision. Cataract.
Pimples and warts on face, and nose.
Articulation of jaws difficult.
Aversion to sweets, likes smoked meat.
Fissures in anus. Fistula and Haemorrhoids.
Involuntary urination on coughing and sneezing.
Retention of urine after surgery.
Uterine inertia. Menstrual flow only during day.
Sudden loss of voice. Vocal cord paralysis; Aphonia. Ch.hoarseness in singers and public speakers.
Cough, with rawness in chest, better drinking cold water.
Gradual loss of muscular power. Gradual paralysis.
Stiffness in back.
Contracture of muscles and tendons.
Rheumatic tearing in limbs, better by heat.
Convulsions and cramps. Epilepsy in young persons.
Gradually increasing hysteria.
Large warts bleed easily, old scars and cicatrices freshen up.
Burns and scalds,

Modalities: Worse dry, cold winds, in clear fine weather, cold air, from motion of carriage, fright, grief or sorrow, suppressed eruptions.
Better damp, wet weather, warmth, heat of bed.

Dosage : 30 th in all conditions, higher in nervous conditions, Paralysis etc.

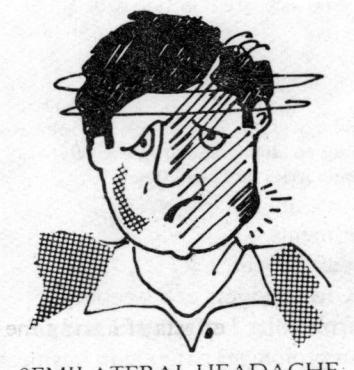

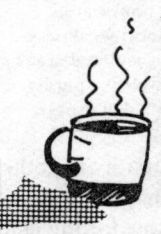

TOOTHACHE:
WORSE:
HEAT, COFFEE

SEMILATERAL HEADACHE
AND THROBBING TOOTHACHE:

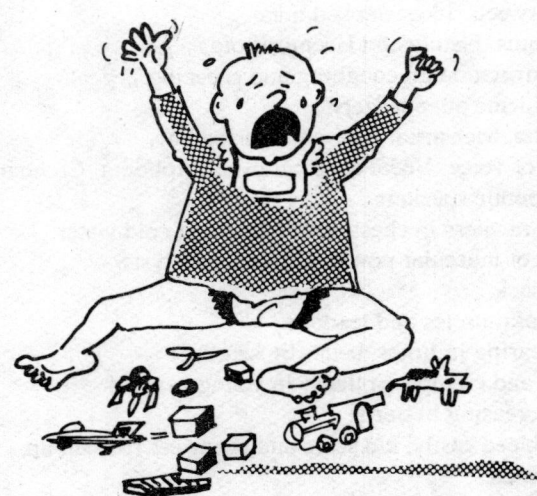

CHILD IRRITABLE, CRIES AND CRIES,
QUIET ONLY WHEN CARRIED

CHAMOMILLA

Common name Matricaria chamomilla. N.O. compositae. Tincture of whole fresh plant.

Pathogenetic sphere of action
- Hyperaesthesia to pain with feeling of numbness
- Digestive disorders.
- Patient is irritable easily angered, moody, and hateful.

Sensitiveness, unquenchable thirst, numbness, irritability and heat.
Hypersensitive to pains.
Great restlessness. Piteous moaning.
Complaints from contradiction, from anger.
Quarrelsome, easily excited to anger. Bad effects of having the feelings wounded.
Never satisfied, wants something new every minute and refuses when offered.
Child always wants to be carried.
Congestive headache, violent earache.
Facial neuralgia.
Toothache from warm drink , from cold air; better cold liquids.
Gums swollen and inflamed. Threatened abscess of gums.
Teeth feels too long- Peridontitis.
Violent flatulent colic, especially in infants.
Colic while urinating.
Grassgreen stools or like chopped eggs.
Dysmenorrhoea, especially following anger.
Tickling cough with rawness in larynx.
Auxious dreams, sees horrible things.

Modalities: Worse by heat, anger, open air, wind, night. Better from being carried, warm wet weather.

Dosage : 12th twice daily.

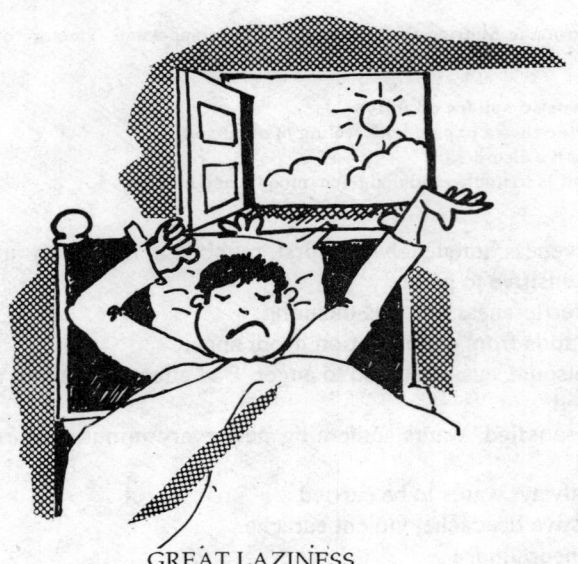

GREAT LAZINESS

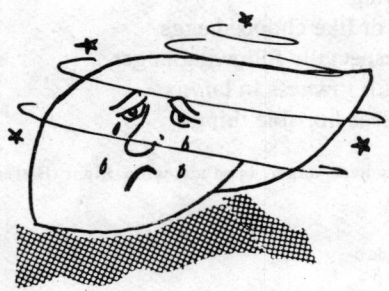

LIVER AND GALLBLADDER AILMENTS

CHELIDONIUM MAJUS

Common name greater celandine. N.O. Papaveraceae. Tincture of entire fresh plant, at time of flowering.

Pathogenetic sphere of action
- Digestive tract especially on liver causing hypertrophy with pain in right hypochondrium This pain radiates up to the lower corner of the right shoulder blade.

An excellent remedy for various liver disorders.
Complaints originated primarily or associated with liver are covered by this drug.
Great laziness and lethargy.
Head feels heavy. Right sided headache with neuralgia over right eye.
Face yellow, jaundiced look.
Eyes- dirty, yellow colour of palpaberal conjunctive.
Tongue yellow and coated.
Prefers hot food and liquids.
Anorexia, eating relieves for short time.
Gall bladder colic. Chronic cholecystitis.
Jaundice   due to hepatic diseases. Liver enlarged.
Urine yellow, foamy and profuse.
Stools constipated, clay colored or alternating diarrhoea and constipation.
Constant pain in back under inferior angle of right scapula.
Serous effusions e.g. Hydrocele etc.
Chiefly right sided remedy.

Modalities: Worse right side, motion, touch, change of weather, very early in morning.
Better after dinner, from pressure.

Dosage : 6th or 30th few doses daily. 200th or above for neuralgias.

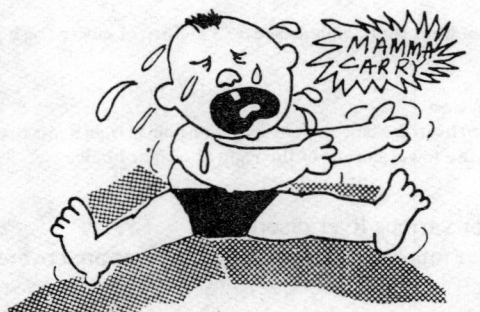

HUNGRY - CROSS-WANTS TO BE CARRIED AND ROCKED

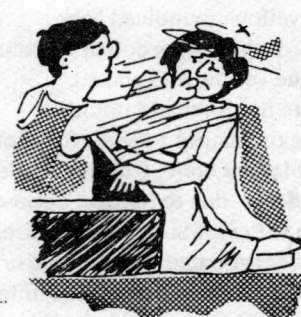

CHILD CRIES AND STRIKES..

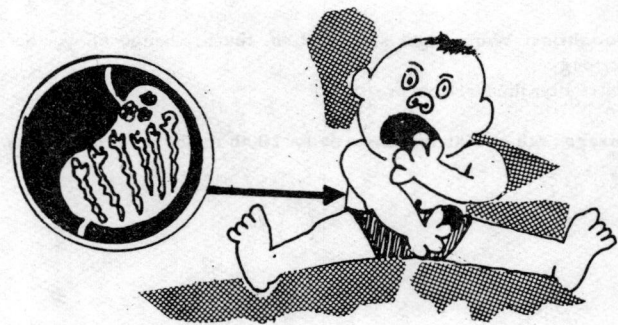

"WORMS", CRAVES SWEET, PICKS THE NOSE.

CINA

Somen cinae. Flores cinae. Artemisia contra. Common name Worm seed. N.O. Compositae.
Tincture of whole plant.

Pathogenetic sphere of action
- The gastrointestinal system causing symptoms usually associated with Intestinal parasites.
- Nervous system to counteract the poisionous effects of loxin liberated by worms.

The child exceedingly cross, wants to be carried and kept busy.

Child wants something, but does not know what, is aggravated by touch and even by being looked at.

Kicks and strikes at the attendant, can not have the hair combed.

Congestive headache relieved by rollling the head.

Symptoms of eye strain, all sorts of colours before the eyes, especially yellow.

Strabismus when worms are present.

Face sunken, Pale, blue rings around eyes and mouth.

Child rubs its nose with the hands or on the pillow, or on the mother's shoulder.

Child bores into the nose until the blood comes.

Grinding of teeth during sleep.

Canine hunger; desire for sweets; refuses mother's milk.

Abdomen bloated and hard, twisting pain around navel.

Child will flop over on its belly and get to sleep in that way.

Itching of anus at night. Child discharges worms.

Urine turns milky on standing.

Whooping cough ends in a spasm.

Twitching and jerking of fingers of right hand.

Stool is not very copious, and often white.

Over sensitiveness to touch.

Modalities: Worse looking fixedly at one object, from worms, at night, sun, in summer.

Dosage : 200th or higher. Weekly for worms.

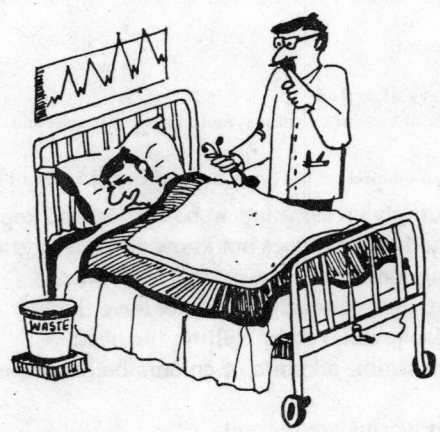

LOW FORM OF FEVERS- MALARIAL FEVER

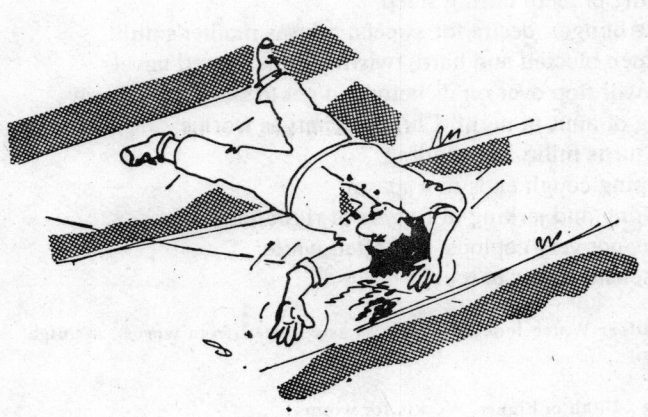

AILMENTS-LOSS OF BLOOD-FOLLOWING

CINCHONA OFFICINALIS

Cinchona calisaya. Common name Peruvian bark. N.O. Rubiaceae. Tincture of dried bark.

Pathogenetic sphere of action

- The ears causing ringing accompained by hypersensitivity of the senses.
- The gastro intestinal system causing flatulence and diarrhoea.
- The circulartory system causing hypotension with dizziness, headaches, cardiac weakness and collapse.

Complaints following the loss of blood and other animal fluids.
Gradually increasing sensitivity to external impressions.
Marked periodicity.
Bleeding tendency.
Chronic liver disorders with jaundice, especially in the persons who are living under the effects of malaria.
General aggravation after eating.
Weakness of mind, inability to think or remember, indifferent, low spirited, disinclined to think, building castles in the air.
Insomnia after haemorrhage. Dizziness, fainting and vertigo may be the consequences of haemorrhage.
Congestive headaches, better by hard pressure.
Face withered, shrunken, pale and anaemic.
Great thirst before the chill.
Loss of appetite or canine hunger.
Gastric symptoms from eating fish, fruits and drinking wine.
Great distension of whole abdomen with loud and strong eructations, giving no relief.
Hiccough, nausea vomiting of bile, sour mucus or blood.
Acidity; complaints of stomach after milk.
Chronic diarrhoea with emaciation.
Low forms of wasting fever, remittent or intermittent or malarial.

Modalities: Worse slightest touch, draught of air, every other day, loss of vital fluids, at night, after eating, bending over. Better bending double, hard pressure, open air, warmth.

Dosage : 30th few doses daily lower or Q for tonic action.

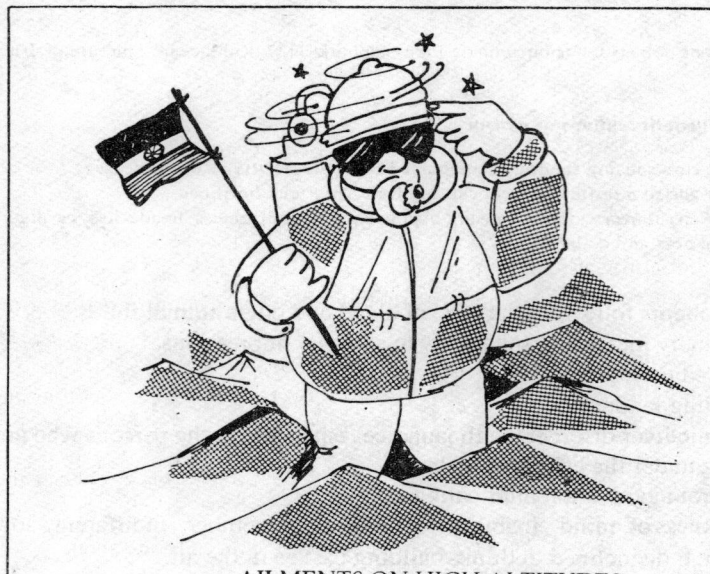

- AILMENTS ON HIGH ALTITUDES
COMPLAINTS OF MOUNTAINEERS

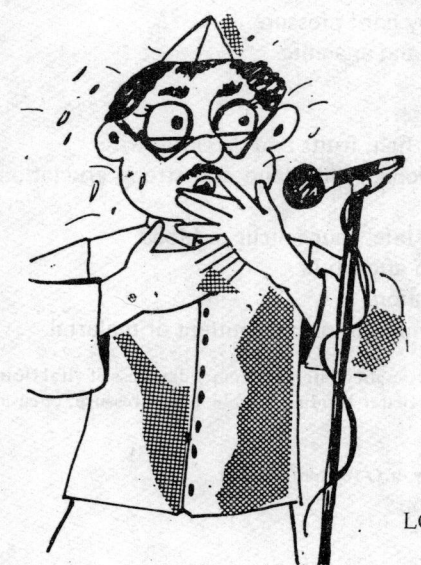

LOSS OF VOICE

COCA-ERYTHROXYLON COCA

N.O. Lineae (suborder Erythroxy leae) Tincture of leaves. Solution or trituration of the alkaloid, Cocaine.

Pathogenetic sphere of action
- The Heart
- The respiratory mucosa.
- The Skin

The mountaineer's remedy.
Complaints developing on climbing mountain e.g. dyspnoea, palpitation, anxiety, insomnia etc.
Loss of voice after talking.
Noises in the ears; headache at high altitude. Emphysema; breathlessness.
Insomnia; sleepy but find no rest anywhere.

Modalities: Worse ascending, high altitudes.Better from wine, riding, quick motion in open air.

Dosage : 30th few doses during acclamtizing as well as on climbing. 200th before use of voice.

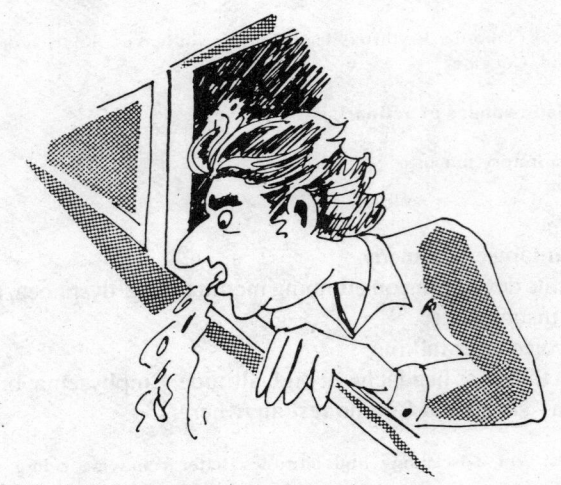

VERTIGO, NAUSEA WHILE TRAVELLING IN A CARRIAGE
" TRAVEL SICKNESS"

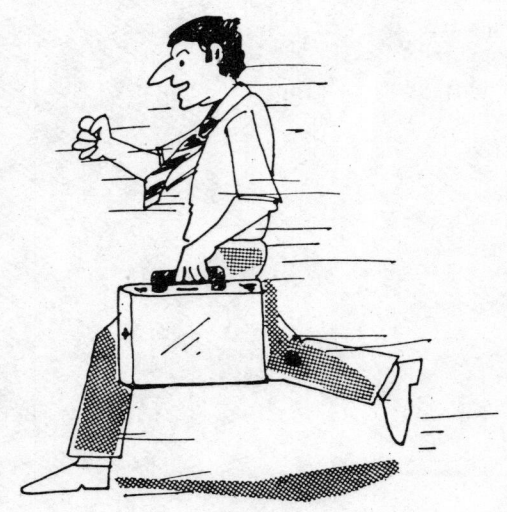

"HURRIED" TIME PASSES TOO QUICKLY

COCCULUS INDICUS

N.O. Menispermaceae. Tincture is prepared from the powdered seeds which contain a crystallisable principle Picrotoxine. a powerful poison.

Pathogenetic sphere of action
- The Cerebro spinal system causing paralytic weakness in motor nerves.
- The Digestive system causing nausea and vomiting with impression of violent dizziness.
- The female genital system causing spasmodic dysmenorrhoea.

Time passes too quickly. Profound sadness.
Vertigo and nausea, especially when riding, travelling and sitting with sense of empitness in head.
Sick headache from travelling.
Cramping pain in masseter muscle.;worse opening mouth. Nausea from riding in bus, car etc., looking at vehicle in motion.
Aversion to food, drug, tobacco, metallic taste.
Smell of food disgusts; desires cold drinks esp. beer.
Sensation of sharp stones filling and moving in stomach.
Weak abdominal muscles.
Dysmenorrhoea and leucorrhoea, very weakening. -
Paralytic pain in small of back.
Pain in shoulder and arms as if bruised.
Trembling in limbs; incoordination of movemnet; locomotor ataxia.
Knees crack on motion; Inflammatory swelling of knee,
Bad effects of night watching.

Modalities: Worse eating, after loss of sleep, open air, smoking, riding, swimming, touch, noise, jar, afternoon, menstural period, after emotional disturbance.

Better good sleep

Dosage : 30th few doses.

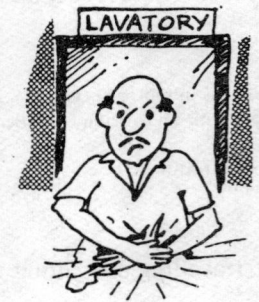

AUTUMN DYSENTERY
WITH VIOLENT TENESMUS

GOUT, ACUTE RHEUMATISM
KNEES STRIKE TOGETHER:
CAN HARDLY WALK

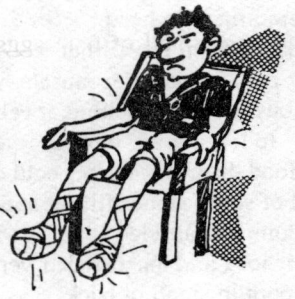

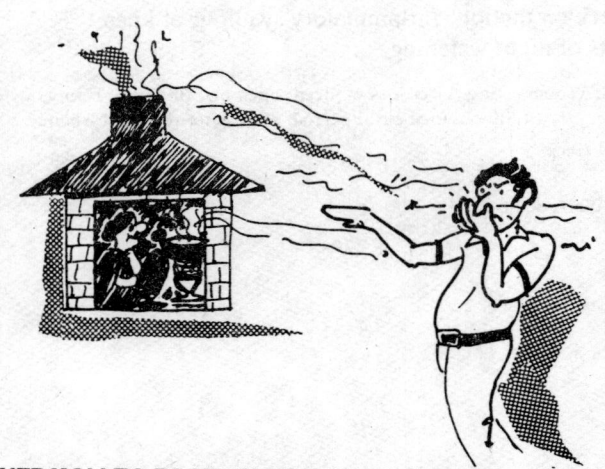

AVERSION TO FOOD (SMELL OF COOKING NAUSEATES)

COLCHICUM AUTUMNALE

Colchium Autumnale. Meadow saffron. N.O. Melanthaceae of the liliaceae.
Tincture of the bulb during spring.

Pathogenetic sphere of action
- The nervous system causing a state of general prostration.
- The digestive mucosa causing a large amounts of diarrhoea and flatulence.
- The articulatory synovial membranes particularly in uric diathesis.

Can read, but cannot understand the words.

Sensitive to noise, light, strong smells etc.

Violent nausea, the thought and smell of food bring on nausea and vomiting.

Aversion to food; smell of fish, eggs, meats, cause nausea even unto faintness.

Violent retching followed by copious and forcible vomiting of food, and then of bile.

Burning in the pit of the stomach.

Abdomen is violently distended and tympanitic.

Grinding of teeth; teeth sensitive when pressed together.

Dysentery in hot, damp weather or in the autumn with white mucus and violent tenesmus.

Bloody discharges from the bowels with deathly nausea.

Acute form of Bright's disease, urine scanty with tenesmus.

Muscular rheumatism and rheumatism of white fibrous tissues of the joints.

Paralytic pains in the arm; and large finger joints. Weakness so that he strikes the knees together when walking.

Swelling of the joints. Gout, complaints are aggravated in cold,damp weather. Complaints are erratic, changing about from place to place.

They are worse from motion and are better by heat, wrapping up.

Profuse and constant sweating.

Modalities: Worse sundown to sunrise, motion, loss of sleep, smell of food in evening, mental exertion. Better stooping.

Dosage : 30th or higher few doses.

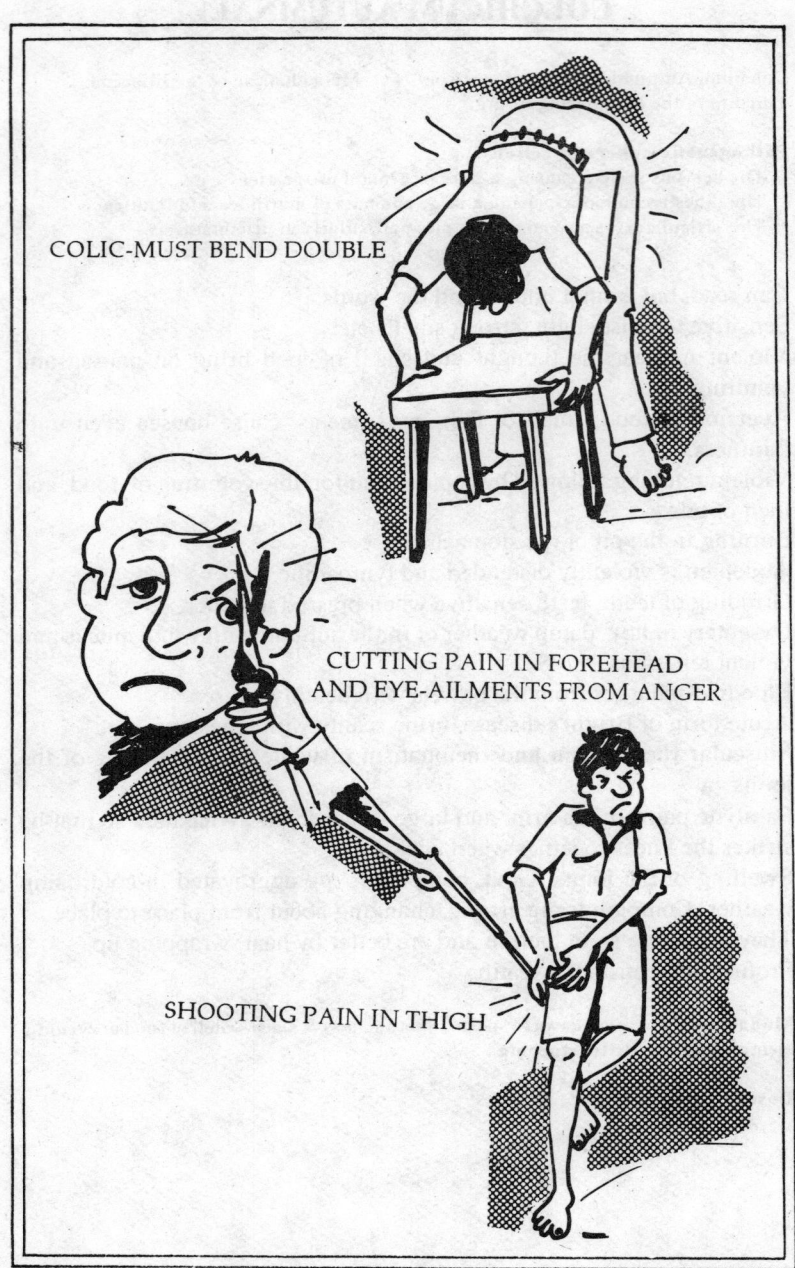

COLIC-MUST BEND DOUBLE

CUTTING PAIN IN FOREHEAD
AND EYE-AILMENTS FROM ANGER

SHOOTING PAIN IN THIGH

COLOCYNTHIS CUCUMIS

Citrullus colocynthis, bitter Apple. N.O. Cucurbilaceae.
Tincture of pulp of fruit.

Pathogenetic sphere of action
- The spasmodic and paroxysmal pain in digestive and female genital system.
- Paroxysmal neuralgia particularly in trigeminal, femoral and sciatic nerves.

Severe, tearing, neuralgic pains, better from bending double.

Complaints from anger with indignation

Pains come in waves, are better from heat and pressure.

The expression of the anxiety from the severity of the suffering is always on the face of this patient.

Aversion to food, violent thirst; potatoes and starchy food disagrees, colic from drinking while overheated.

Violent griping in the umbilical region, obliging the patient to bend double.

Nausea and vomiting occurs due to violence of pain.

Diarrhoea and dysentery from anger.

Eating little, brings on the colic and urging for stool.

Violent shooting pain in the right thigh, worse on walking.

Sciatica, of left side, better by pressure and heat.

Modalities: Worse from anger, indignation. Better doubling up, hard pressure, warmth, lying with head bent forward.

Dosage : 30th in gastric complaints, frequently. 200th or higher for neuralgias.

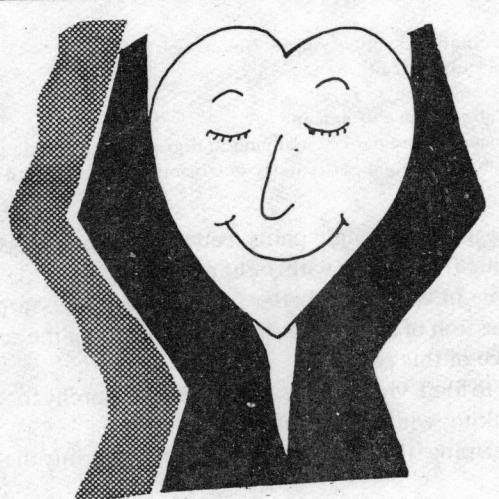

HEART TONIC

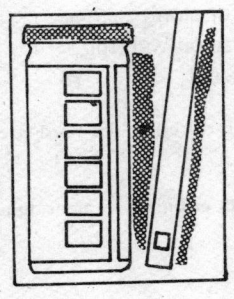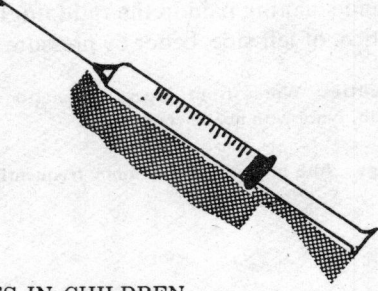

DIABETES IN CHILDREN

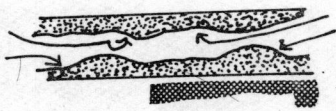

ATHEROSCLEROSIS

CRATAEGUS OXYCANTHA

Crataegus oxyacantha. Hawthorn. N.O. Rosaceae.
Tincture of ripe fruit.

Pathogenetic sphere of action
- The Heart.
- The blood vessels esp. arteries.

It is a heart tonic.
Irregularity of heart.
Arteriosclerosis : said to have a solvent power upon crustaceous and calcareous deposits in arteries.
Diabetes especially in Children.
Cardiac dropsy.
Extreme dyspnoea on least exertion, without much increase of pulse.
Pain in region of heart and under left clavide
Heart dilated, first sound weak.
Pulse accelerated irregular feeble, intermittent

Modalities: Worse in warm room. Better fresh air, quiet, rest.

Dosage : Q or 3x few doses daily. Wait for its tonic efferts to be evident.

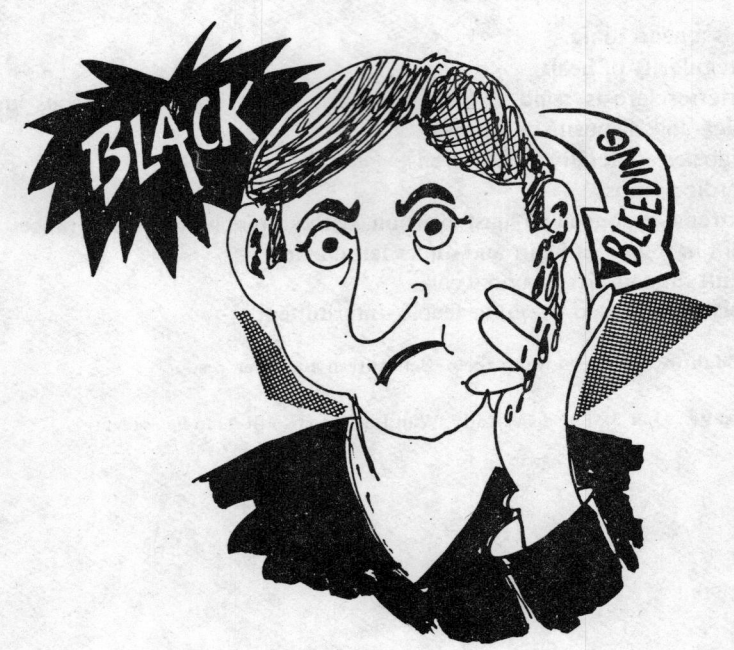

"HAEMORRHAGES' DARK AND BLACK

CROTALUS HORRIDUS

Rattle Snake. N.O.Crotalidae. Trituration of sugar of milk saturated with the venom. Solution of the venom in glycerine.

Pathogenetic sphere of action
- The nervous system.
- The circulatory system
- The blood causing haemorrhages.

Haemorrhagic tendency. Haemolysis. Yellow fever.
Haemorrhages dark, no clot formation.
Sleeps into the symptoms.
Right sidedness.
Loquacious with desire to escape.
Headache; must walk on tip toe to avoid jarring.
Very sensitive to light, especially lamp light.
Ciliary neuralgia, absorbs intraocualr haemorrhages.
Black blood oozes from ears.
Epistaxis, blood black stringy.
Black or coffee ground vomiting.
Cancer of stomach with haematemesis black.
Gastritis in chronic alcoholics.
Malaena: intestinal haemorrhage. Blood dark, fluid non-coagulable.
Haemoptysis.
Right sided paralysis.
Yellow fever. Purpura haemorrhagica.
Dreams of dead.

Modalities: Worse right side, open air, evening and morning, in spring, coming on of warm weather, on awaking, damp and wet, jar.

Dosage : 30th repeatedly for hges. 200th or higher for paralysis.

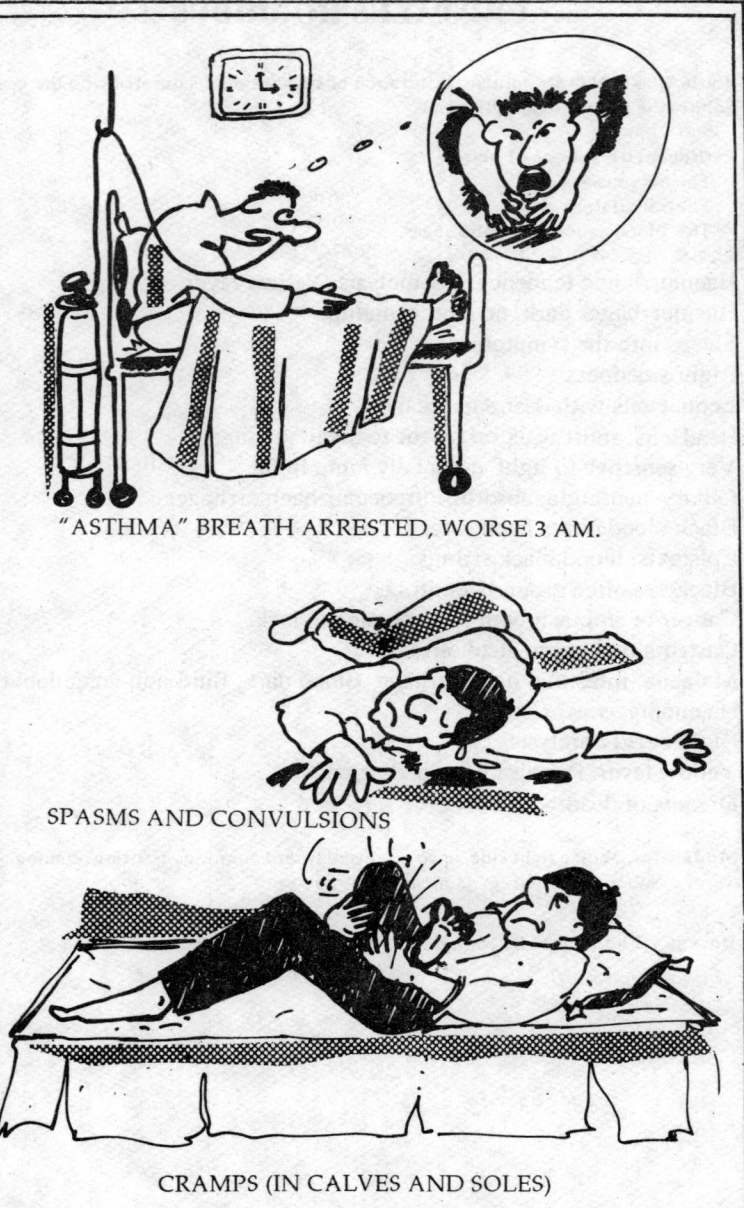

"ASTHMA" BREATH ARRESTED, WORSE 3 AM.

SPASMS AND CONVULSIONS

CRAMPS (IN CALVES AND SOLES)

CUPRUM METALLICUM

Copper Cu(A.W.63) Trituration.

Pathogenetic sphere of action
- Spasmodic phenomena in smooth and striated muscles
- Gastro -enteritis.

Spasms; spasmodic affections in general.
Tonic convultion -Epilepsy, beginning in fingers and toes and spreading all over.
Epilepsy; aura begins in knees, with clenched thumbs.
Convulsions with biting.
Spasms followed by the appearance as if the patient was dead.
Complaints from fright and chiefly of left side.
Epilepsy, face blue, contraction of jaws, with foam at mouth.
Eruptive fevers with violent vomiting, stupor, convulsions etc.
Violent contractive pains.
Meningitis.
Strong metalllic taste in mouth with flow of saliva.
Protrusion of tongue like as of a snake.
Nausea. When drinking, the fluid descends with gurgling sound.
Abdominal colic.
Tape worms.
Uraemic convulsions.
Cholera- with cramps in abdomen and calves.
Angina pectoris, precordial anxiety and pain, whooping cough, better drinking water.
Spasmodic Asthma; worse 3 a.m.
Clutches throat with hands, unable to speak or swallow.
Spasms and constriction of chest.
Cramps in calves and soles.

Modalities: Worse before menses, from vomiting, contact. Better during perspiration, drinking cold water.

Dosage : 30th few doses daily.

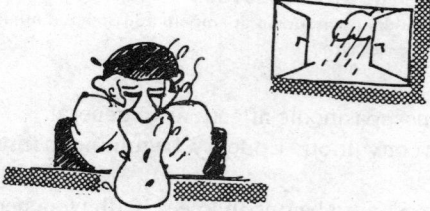

COMPLAINTS AGGRAVATED IN DAMP WEATHER

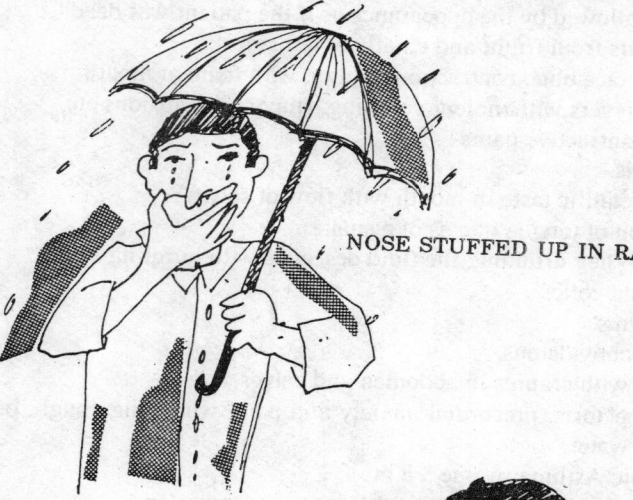

NOSE STUFFED UP IN RAIN

WARTS ON FACE AND PALM

DULCAMARA

Woody nightshade Bitter sweet N.O. solanaceae. Tincture prepared from fresh green stems and leaves, gathered just before flowering.

Pathogenetic sphere of action
- The respiratory and digestive mucosa.
- The lymphatic system causing sudden swelling of lymph nodes.
- The fibro muscular system causing rheumatic pain.
- The skin.

There is alternation between eruptions, diarrhoea and rheumatic symptoms.

The rheumatic troubles induced by damp cold are aggravated by every cold change and relieved by moving about.

Scaldhead, thick brown crusts, bleeding when scratched.

Nose is stuffed up when there is cold rain.

Tearing in cheek extending to ear, orbit and jaw preceded by coldness of parts and attended by canine hunger.

Facial neuralgia worse slightest exposure to cold.

Aversion to food, burning thirst for cold drinks.

Cutting pain about navel.

Must urinate when getting chilled, urine has thick, mucous, purulent sediment.

Before appearance of menses, a rash appears on skin.

Cough after physical exertion.

Pain in small of back as after long stooping.

Paralysis, feet icy cold.

Adenitis. Pruritus always worse in cold wet weather.

Modalities: Worse at night, from cold in general, damp rainy weather. Better from moving about, external warmth.

Dosage : 30th few doses a day.

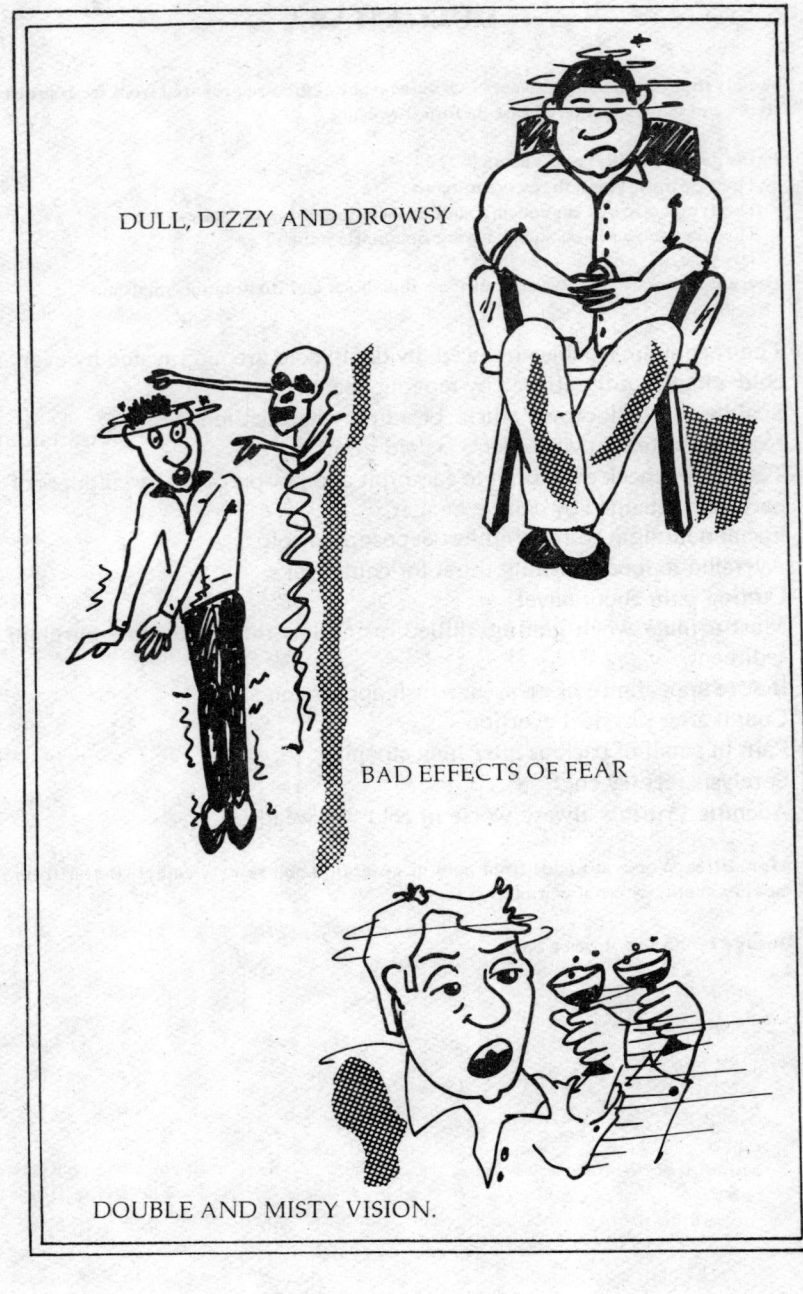

DULL, DIZZY AND DROWSY

BAD EFFECTS OF FEAR

DOUBLE AND MISTY VISION.

GELSEMIUM SEMPERVIUM

Commonly called gelsemium semperivirens. G.Lucidum. G.Nitidum. Bignonia sempervirens.
Common name Yellow Jesamine N.O. loganiaceae.
Tincture of bark of the root.

Pathogenetic sphere of action
- The cerebro spinal system producing initial stage of excitation, trembling, cramps, co-ordination problems.
- It has second paretic phase due to passive congestion causing general prostration and heaviness.
- The circulation system, causing slowing down of heart beat and hypotension.
- The respiratory and digestive mucosa causing catarrhal inflammation.

Dullenss, dizziness and drowsiness.
Motor paralysis. Muscular paralysis, lack of muscular co-ordination; trembling.
Insidious development of complaints.
Post-diphtheric paralysis.
Incapacity to think, or fix the attention.
Anticipation brings on diarrhoea.
Complaints from embarrassment; from fright or shock.
Most violent occipital headache preceded by blindness and better by profuse urination.
Vertigo.
Droping of eyelids (Ptosis).
Double and misty vision. Orbital neuralgia.
Complete thirstlessness.
Partial paralysis of bladder.
Feels it was necessary to keep in motion or heart' would cease beating.
Weak, slow pulse, palpitation.
Complete relaxation of whole muscular system, great heaviness of the limbs. Numbness and tingling in fingers and palms.
Nervous chills, wants to be held, because he shakes so violently.
Chilliness along spine.
Influenza.
Measles with catarrhal symptoms.
Sleep greatly disturbed.

Modalities: Worse damp weather, fog, before a thunderstorm, emotion, excitement, bad news, tobacco smoking, when thinking of his ailments, 10 a.m. Better Bending forward, by profuse urination, open air, continued motion, stimutants.

Dosage : 6th or 30th in acute complaints. 200th or higher in neurological ailments.

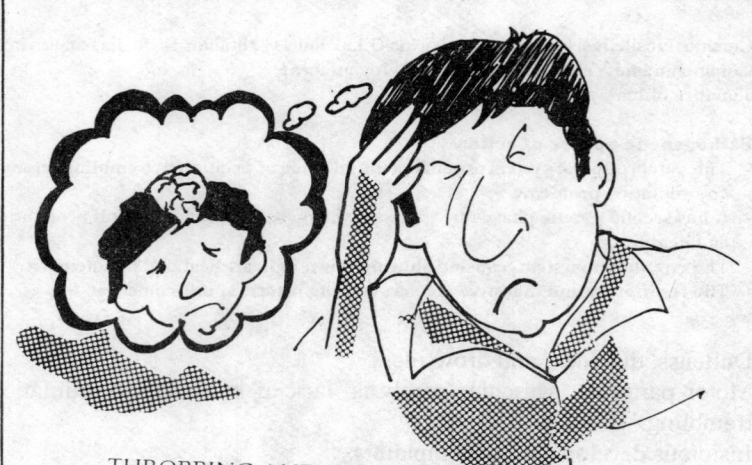

THROBBING AND BURSTING HEADACHE

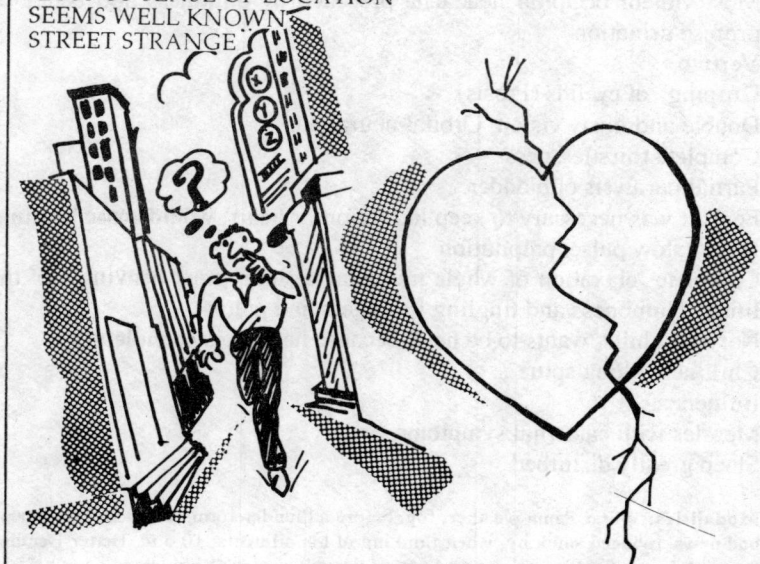

PALPITATION AND ANGINA

GLONOINUM

Nitro glycerine $C_3H_5(NO_3)O_3$. Dilutions with alcohol.

Pathogenetic sphere of action
- Circulatory erythism with palpitations
- Brutal, violent cephalic congestion.
- There is alternate periods of vasodilation and vasoconstriction.

Mental confusion. Loss of sense of location. Well known streets seem strange.
Congestive headache. Cerebrospinal meningitis.
Throbbing in temples, in front of head; as if blood was surging to head; as if skull was too small and brain attempting to burst it.
SUNSTROKE. Headache increases and decreases with SUN.
SEASICKNESS. ANGINA PECTORIS
Bad effects from mental excitement, fright, from exposure to sun rays, gas light etc.
Epileptic convulsions, clenching and jerking upwards of fist and legs.
Violent palpitation with throbbing carotids.
Laborious action of heart; pulse quick and irregular.
Bad effects of old contusions and concussions; having hair cut.
Sensation of pulsation throughout body.

Modalities: Worse in sun, exposure to sun rays, gas, open fire, jar, stooping, having hair cut, peaches, stimulants, lying down, from 6 a.m. to noon, left side. Better brandy, in dark, cool atmosphere.

Dosage : 3x frequently brings down blood pressure quickly, reduces coronary and cerebral insufficiency.

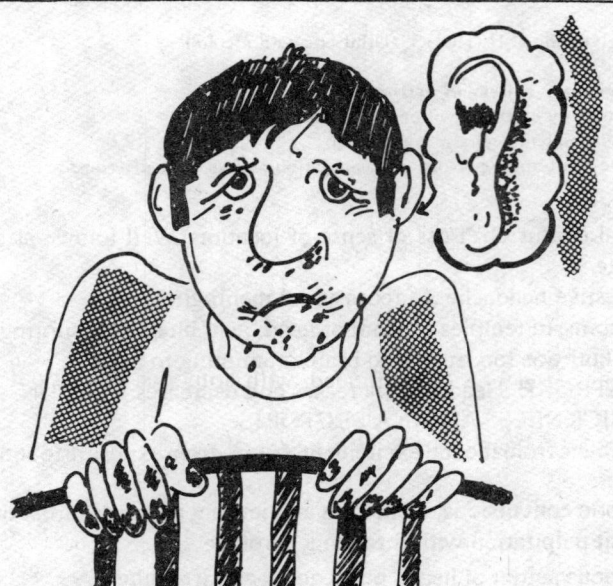

BLEPHARITIS, MOIST CRACKS BEHIND EAR
"ECZEMATOUS ERUPTIONS"
ULCERATED NOSTRILS AND LIPS, BAD NAILS

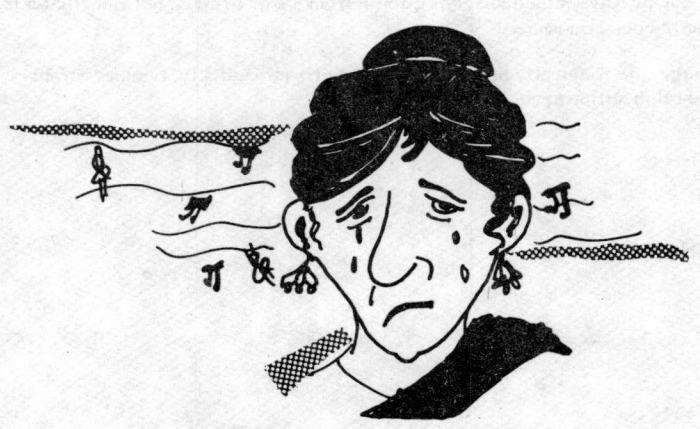

DEPRESSED, MUSIC MAKES HER WEEP

GRAPHITES

Plumbago. Black lead. It is an allotropic modification of carbon. Trituration of prepared black lead from fine English drawing pencils.

Pathogenetic sphere of action
- The skin causing suppurating eczematous eruptions.
- The digestive tract causing atony and flatulence.
- The genital organs causing slowing down of utero-ovarian functions and lack of sex-drive.
- The circulatory system causing anaemia and tendency to haemorrhage.

Tendency to obesity with anaemia. Chilly.

Great sadness. Depression with tendency to weep. Music makes her weep.

Mucous outlets of body inflamed, with eruptions oozing out glutinous discharge.

Falling of hair, eczema capitis, oozing sticky fluid.

Eyes-inflamed margins of lids.

Moist and sore places behind the ears.

Dry scabs in nose, cannot tolerate flowers.

Soreness and cracks of lips and nostrils.

Aversion to fish, meat, etc.

Sweets disagree and nauseate. Hot drinks disagree.

Stomach pains relieved by eating hot food, relieved by lying down.

Duodenal ulcer.

Constipation - stools knotty, covered with mucus.

Greatly distended abdomen; hardness of liver region.

Itching of anus. Haemorrhoids with burning of liver region.

Decided aversion to coitus.

Cancer of mammary glands, cracks in nipples with soreness.

Skin, hard and cracked in several places.

Finger nails brittle, do not grow; become thick and black.

Eruptions, itching and oozing out sticky fluid.

Offensive perspiration of feet.

Every injury suppurates.

Modalities: Worse warmth, at night; during and after mensturation. Better in the dark from wrapping up.

Dosage : 6th in skin ailments (Promises no aggravation) 200th or higher as constitutional.

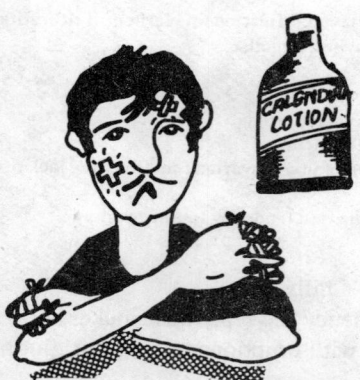

EVERY INJURY SUPPURATES EVEN SLIGHTEST

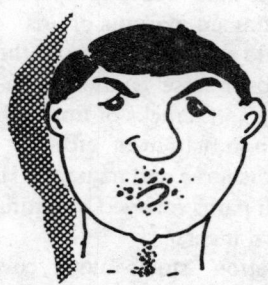

PAIN WITH SPLINTER SENSATION IN THROAT

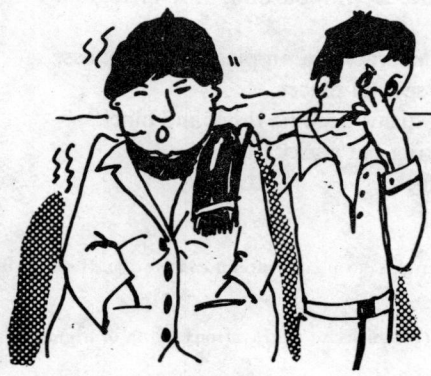

OFFENSIVE SMELL FROM THE BODY.

SENSITIVE TO OPEN AIR. EXTREMELY CHILLY.

HEPAR SULPHURIS

Commonly called sulphuris Calcareum. An impure sulphide of calcium prepared by burning in a crucible the white interior of oyster shells with pure flowers of sulphur. Trituration.

Pathogenetic sphere of action
- The nervous system causing hypersensitivity both mentally and physically.
- It has strong tendency towards inflammation with tendency to suppurate in the mucous membrane expecially of skin, respiratory mucosa particularly the larynx and the lymphatic tissue.

Patient is chilly and hypersensitive to external impressions, especially pain. Potbellied and smelly.

Extreme irriability and over sensitiveness.

Every little thing makes him angry, abusive and impusive e.g. sudden impulse in a barber's mind to cut the throat of his customer while in the chair.

Quarrelsome, hard to be pleased; oversensitiveness to people, and to places.

Extremely chilly; putting the hand or foot out of bed brings a general worsening of all complaints.

Catarrhal state in general, of nose, ear, throat, tongue, chest, etc.

Offensive discharges smell like decomposed cheese.

Child always smell sour inspite of repeated washing.

Tonsils swollen, pain as if from fish bone or splinter in throat.

Profuse sweating all night without relief.

Acute otitis media.

Cattarrhal inflammation of eyes. Stye.

Suffocating cough with sensation of plug in throat. CROUP.

Great desire for vinegar.

Localized inflammations inclined to suppurate, ulcer and eruption are extremely sensitive to touch.

Deep cracks on hand and feet.

Chronic and recurring urticaria.

Pustules spread by coalising.

Modalities: Worse- dry cold winds, cool air, slightest draught, Mercury, touch, lying on painful side. Better, damp weather, from wrapping head up, from warmth, after eating.

Dosage : 3x hastens suppuration. 200th or higher to prevent recuerrance of infection.

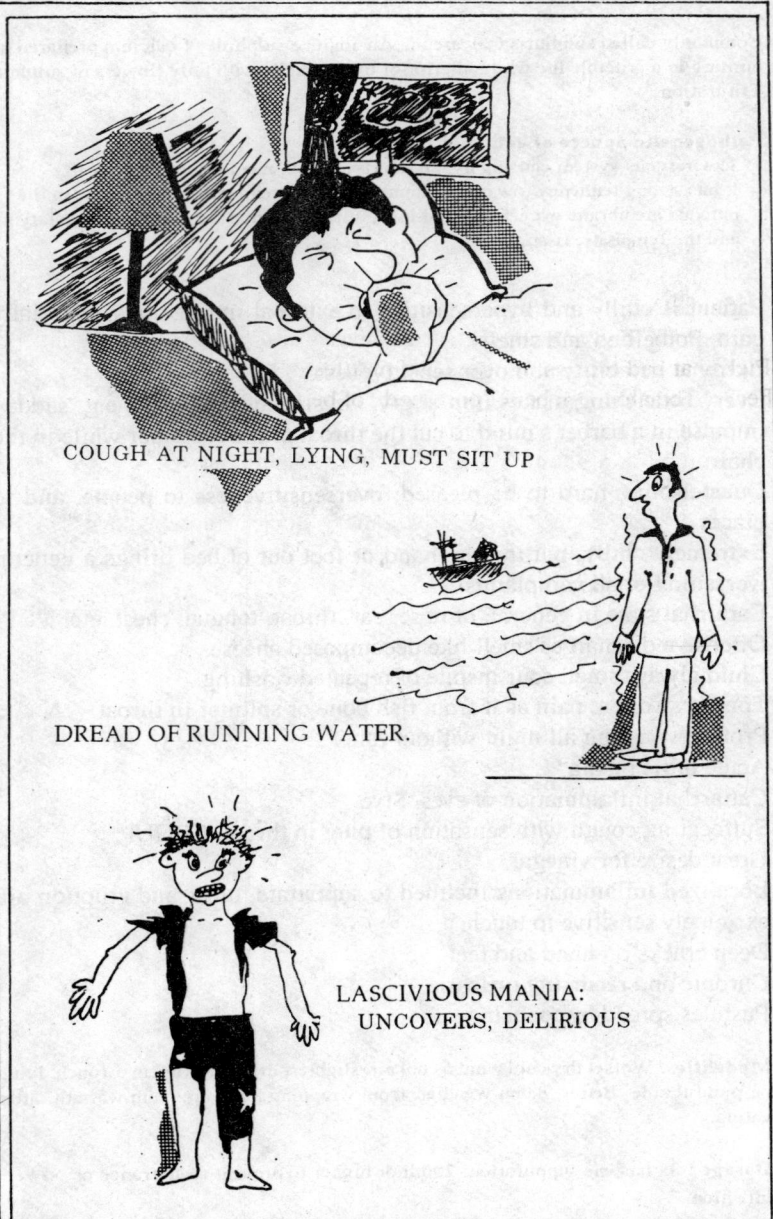

COUGH AT NIGHT, LYING, MUST SIT UP

DREAD OF RUNNING WATER.

LASCIVIOUS MANIA:
UNCOVERS, DELIRIOUS

HYOSCYAMUS NIGER

Common name Henbane. N.O. - Solanaceae. Tincture of fresh plant is prepared.

Pathogenetic sphere of action
- The cerebro-spinal system causing phases of excitation with spasms, asthenic with passive congestion and paralytic with coma.

Convulsion, contractions and violent trembling.
Delirium with restlessness; foolish laughter; silly expressions.
Lascivious mania; uncovers, strips herself naked; sings amorous songs.
Suspicious, jealous with rage and delirium; with attempt to murder.
Picks at bed clothes, mutters and prattles in bed.
Fears to be alone, of being poisoned , of being injured.
Constant carphologia, deep stupor.
Inflammation of brain; vertigo as if intoxicated.
Dread of running water.
Pupils dilated, double vision, involuntary stool, urination.
Dry spasmodic cough, worse lying down.
Convulsions.
EPILEPSY: before attack, vertigo or ringing in ears with cramps in calves and toes.
Great restlessness; every muscle twitches.
Intense sleeplessness, starts up frightened.
Patient will never remain covered.

Modalities: Worse at night during menses, after eating, when lying down. Better stooping.

Dosage : 200th few doses and wait.

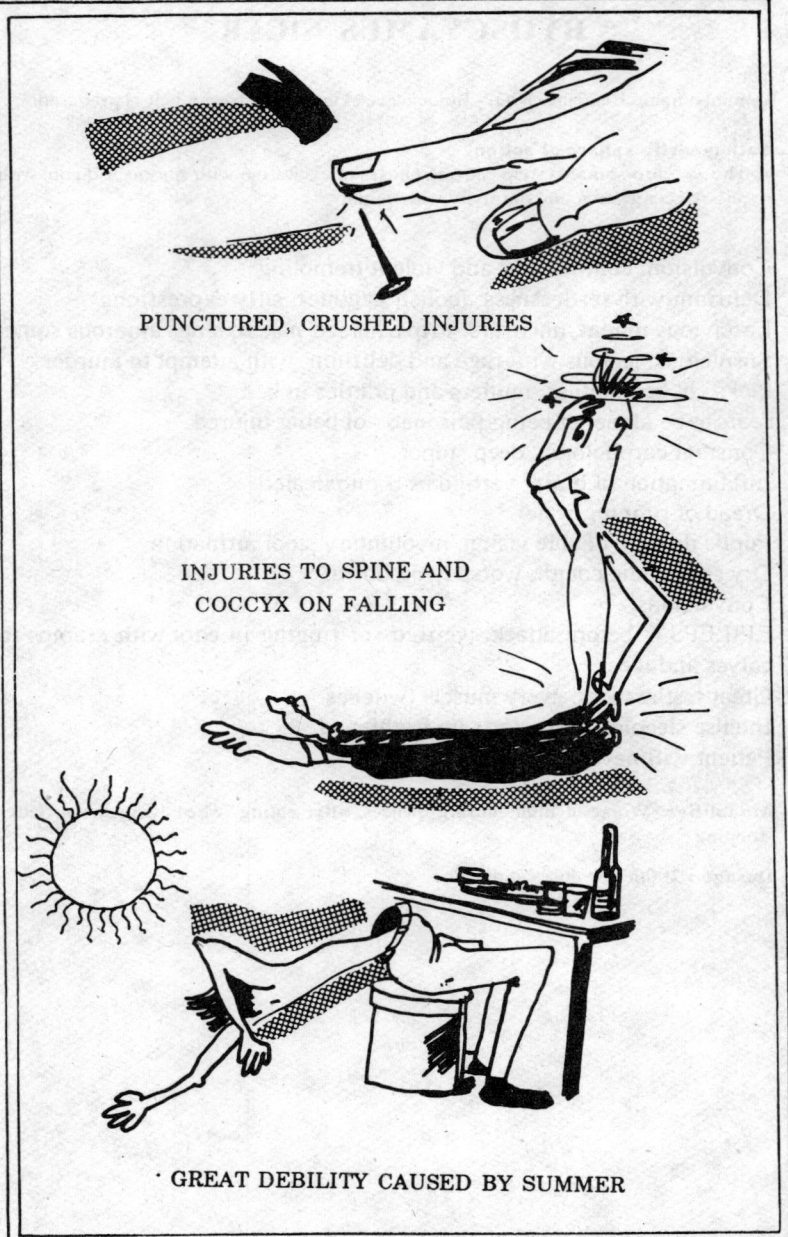

PUNCTURED, CRUSHED INJURIES

INJURIES TO SPINE AND
COCCYX ON FALLING

· GREAT DEBILITY CAUSED BY SUMMER

HYPERICUM PERFORATUM

Hyperium perforatum . St.John's wort. N.O.Hypericaceae. Tincture of whole fresh plant.

Pathogenetic sphere of action
- The nerve endings
- There is traumatism of cerebro spinal system.

Punctured wounds.

Coccydynia.

Head feels heavy as if touched by on icy cold hand.

Throbbing in vertex worse in close room.

Head feels longer elongated to a point.

Nausea.

Haemorrhoids with pain, bleeding and tenderness.

Pressure over sacrum.

Crawling in hand and feet.

Neuritis with tingling,burning pain, numbness and glossy skin.

Asthma worse foggy weather and relieved by profuse perspiration.

Injuries to nerves especially of fingers, toe and nails.

Relieves pain after operations.

Modalities: Worse in cold, dampness, in fog, in close room, least exposure, touch. Better bending head backward.

Dosage : 200th or higher few doses.

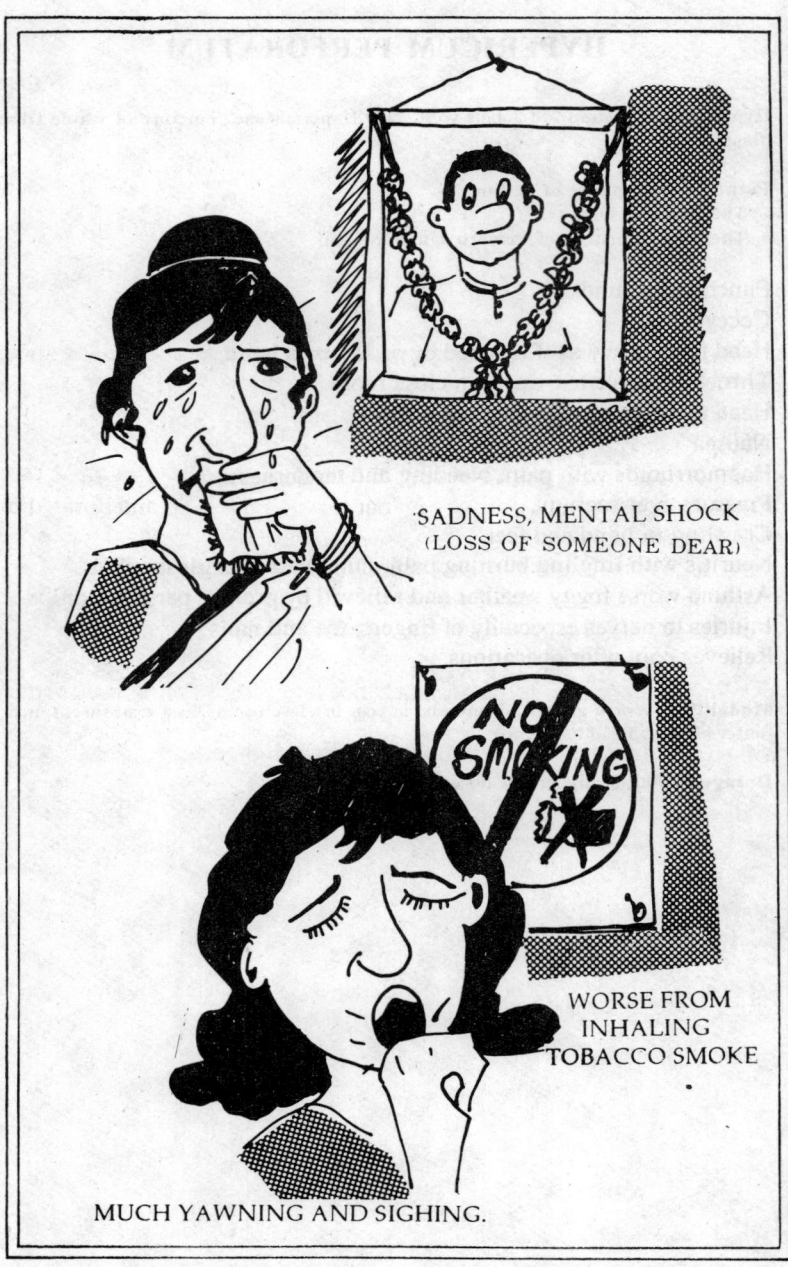

SADNESS, MENTAL SHOCK
(LOSS OF SOMEONE DEAR)

WORSE FROM INHALING TOBACCO SMOKE

MUCH YAWNING AND SIGHING.

IGNATIA AMARA

Common name Faba indica. St.Ignatius Bean. N.O.loganiaceae. Tincture and trituration of the seeds.

Pathogenetic sphere of action
- Marked hyperaesthesia of all organs and senses.
- There is mental hypersensitivity to emotion.
- There is tendency towards various types of spasms.
- There is general inco-ordination of the various organic functions.

Tearful, nervous sad and sensitive women.
Feeling of continous fright or apprehensiveness that something is going to happen.
Great grief after losing persons or objects very dear.
Changeable mood, sighing and sobbing.
Much yawning and great aversion to smoking tobacco.
Headache, as if a nail were driven out through the side; ameliorated by lying upon the side affected.
Headache from abuse of coffee; from inhaling tobacco smoke etc.
Asthenopia, disturbance of vision.
Follicular tonsilitis, pain better by swallowing.
Globus hystericus.
Feeling of emptiness in the stomach, not relieved by eating, relieved by taking a deep breath.
Much flatulence, aversion to food but craves indigestible things.
Prolapse of rectum with stitches in haemorrhoids.
Painful contraction of anus after stool.
Jerking of limbs on falling asleep.
Sleep so light that he hears everything while asleep.
Insomnia from grief.
Thirst during chill but not during the fever.

Modalities: Worse in morning, open air, after meals, coffee, smoking, liquids, external warmth. Better while eating, change of position.

Dosage : 200th few doses.

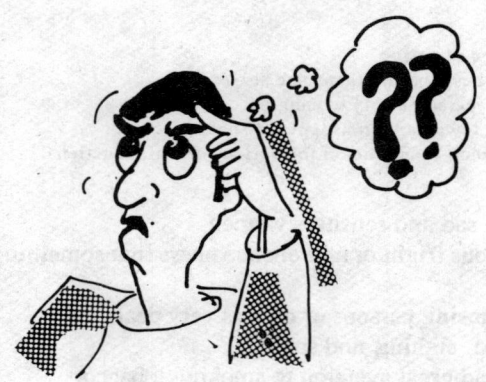

HAS FORGOTTEN SOMETHING: DOES NOT KNOW WHAT

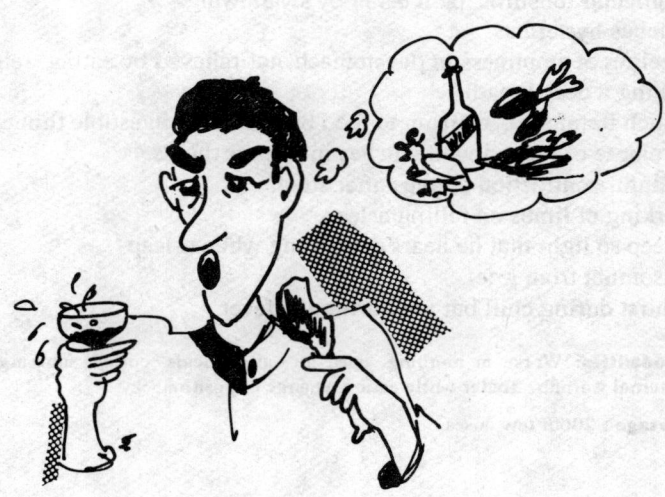

LIKES LIQUOR AND MEAT, GREAT HUNGER (YET LOSES FLESH)

IODUM

Iodine. It is an element I. (A.W. 126-53). Tincture.

Pathogenetic sphere of action
- The mucous membrane causing irritation and formation of pseudo membranes.
- The lymph nodes and endocrine glands causing painless hypertrophy and induration of thyroid, testicles, ovaries, mammary glands, pancreas etc.
- The skin causing red indurated elements like acne.
- It has general effect on nutrition.

Dark haired, dark eyed, dark skinned, warm blooded, impatient persons.
Has forgotten something, but does not know what.
Must be busy whole day and night, never sits down nor sleeps at night.
Vertigo lying on left side, worse stooping.
Goitre. Protrusion of eye balls.
Eats too often and too much, and loses flesh all the while.
Alternate canine hunger and loss of appetite.
Desire for meat and spirituous liquor.
Spleen and liver painful and enlarged; Jaundice.
Atrophy of ovaries and mammary glands with sterility.
Enlargement and induration of glands.
Intolerance of heat.
Sensation as if heart were squeezed by hand.
Hypertrophy of heart.
Chronic arthritic affections with violent pain in joints at night.
Chronic morning diarrhoea of emaciated, scrofulous children.
Suffocating cough. All discharges are, extremely acrid.

Modalities: Worse when quiet, in warm room, right side. Better walking about, in open air.

Dosage : 30th few doses a day.

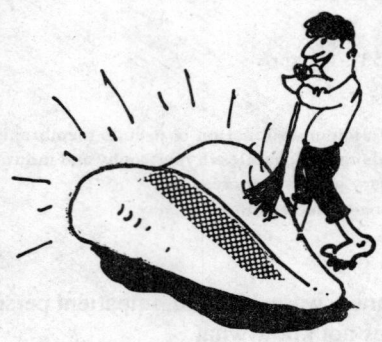

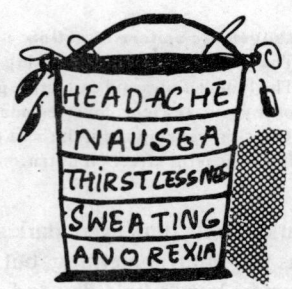

CLEAN TONGUE

BRIGHT RED AND PROFUSE BLEEDING

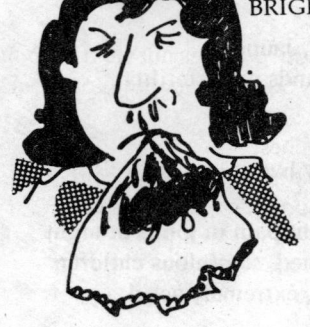

COLIC AROUND NAVEL
(CUTTING, CLUTCHING PAIN)

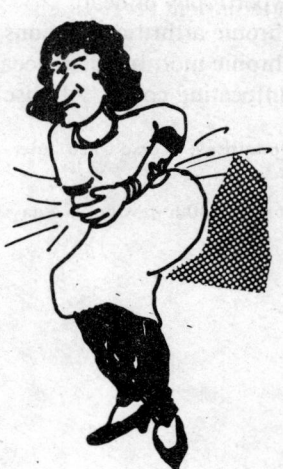

IPECACUANHA

Common name Cephaelis ipecacuanha. N.O. Rubiaceae. Tincture and trituration of the dried root.

Pathogenetic sphere of action
- The digestive tract causing spasmodic, nausea, vomiting and diarrhoea.
- The respiratory tract causing catarrhal inflammation with spasmodic dyspnoea, asthma etc.
- It also causes haemorrhage of bright red blood in both of above tracts.

Persistent nausea and vomiting.

Haemorrhages bright red and profuse.

Tongue usually clean; much saliva, constant nausea and vomiting.

Cutting, clutching pain around navel.

Amoebic dysentery, stool, pitch like, green as grass, like frothy molasses; griping at navel, uterine haemorrhages; profuse, bright gushing with nausea.

Pain from navel to uterus.

Vomiting during pregnancy.

Rattling cough; chest feels full of phelgm, but does not yield to coughing.

Cough incessant and violent, with every breath, whooping cough, nausea.

Haemoptysis.

Asthma with constant constriction of chest.

Hoarseness; complete aphonia, especially at the end of cold.

Intermittent fever- slight chill with much heat and nausea.

Modalities: Worse periodically, from veal, moist warm wind, lying down.

Dosage : 3x frequently in acute gastric complaints.

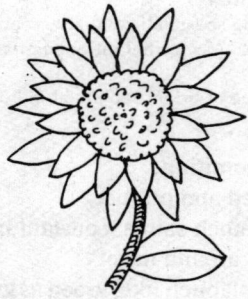

YELLOWNESS

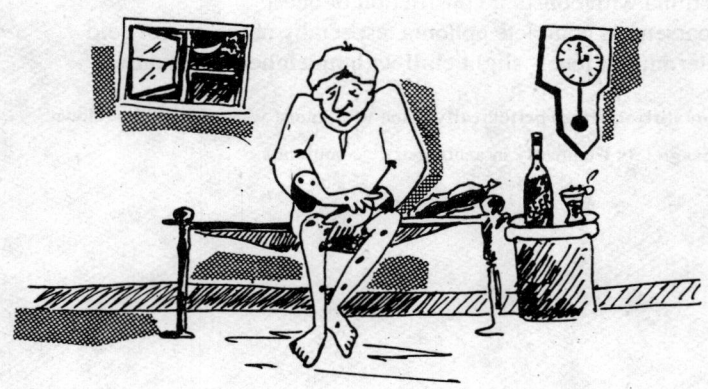

PAIN IN SPOTS - BAD EFFECTS OF BEER- WORSE 2-3 A.M.

KALI BICHROMICUM

Bichromate of Potash $K_2Cr_2O_7$. Solution in distilled water. Trituration.

Pathogenetic sphere of action
- The mucosa particularly of digestive and respiratory tracts causing inflammation with large amounts of mucous secretion which is sticky and forms thick yellow green membranes and formation of deep ulcerations.
- The fibrous tissue and the periosteum causing articular pains and suppuration in the ears.
- The skin causing ulcerations with sharply defined edges.

Sensitive to cold; lack of vital heat, worse hot weather.

Spottiness-severe pain small in spot, that could be covered by the tip of the thumb.

Yellowness, - tongue yellow, eyes yellow, vomiting yellow, all discharges are yellow.

Stringiness - catarrhal conditions of mucous membranes with stringy discharges from nose, ear and saliva etc.

Wandering rheumatic pains from joint to joint.

Rheumatism alternating with diarrhoea or dysentery.

Complaints worse about 2 or 3 a.m.

Supra-orbital, headache. Headache in small spot.

Catarrhal conjunctivitis with stringy discharges.

Perforation of nasal septum, fetid discharge from nose.

Violent sneezing; loss of smell.

Tongue red, shining and dry.

Nausea and vomiting of beer drinkers.

Ulceration of stomach.

Dislikes meat.

Craves beer which makes him sick.

After urination a drop seems to remain which cannot be expelled.

Metallic cough; with profuse, yellow, stringy expectoration.

Whooping cough.

Pain in coccyx.

Ulcers with punched out edges.

Modalities: Worse beer, morning, hot weather, undressing. Better from heat.

Dosage : 30th repeatedly in gastritis and cough. 200th or higher in rheumatism.

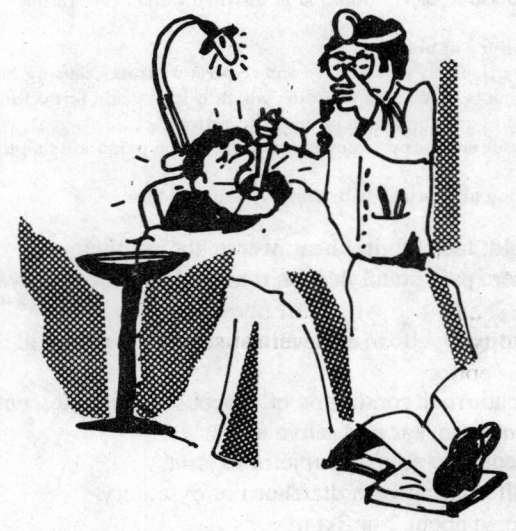

FETID BREATH - GUMS INFLAMED - DENTAL CARIES

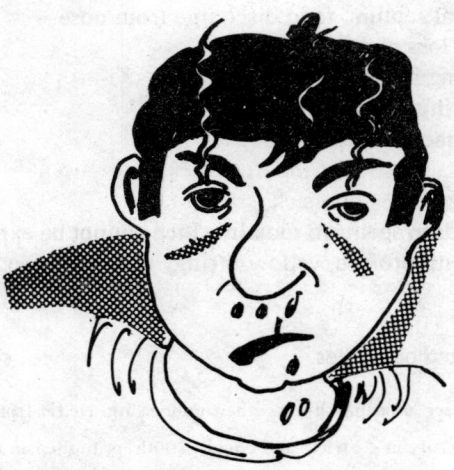

ACRID LACHRYMATION (EXCORIATING DISCHARGES)

KREOSOTUM

Commonly called Kreasote or Creasote. A product of distillation of wood tar. $C_8H_{10}O_2$, solution in Rectified spirit.

Pathogenetic sphere of action
- The mucosa causing inflammation leading to ulceration or necrosis with formation of foetid, burning, corrosive, yelowish white mucopus.
- There is tendency to haemorrhage.

Excoriating discharges, pulsations all over the body.
Profuse bleeding from small wounds.
Every emotion is attended with tearfulness.
Marked irritability in children, never satisfied.
Music causes weeping.
Acrid, salty lachrymation.
Very painful dentition.
Very rapid decay of teeth; teeth dark, crumbling.
Gums- bleeding and spongy, detached.
Fetid odour from mouth.
Appetite increased especially for meat; craves smoked meat.
Vomiting of food several hours after eating.
Haematemesis.
Cholera infantum.
Urine offensive; must hurry when desire comes to urinate.
Nocturnal enuresis; dreams of urinating.
Leucorrhoea, excoriating, yellow, putrid.
Hoarse cough with profuse mucopurulent expectoration.
Gangrene of lungs.
Heaviness, stiffness, numbness, crawling and itching.

Modalities: Worse in open air, cold, rest, when lying, after mensturation. Better from warmth, motion, warm diet.

Dosage : 200th, 1 or 2 doses a day.

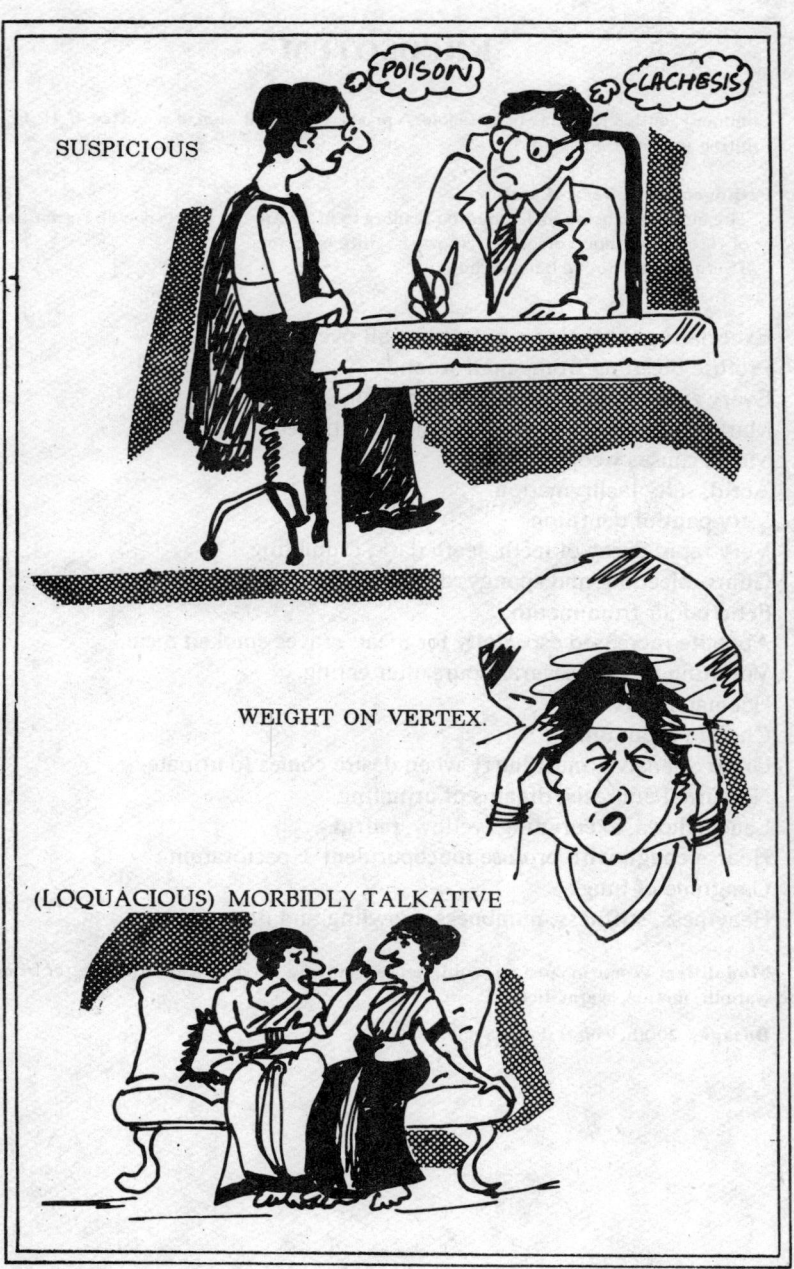

LACHESIS

Trigonocephalus lachesis. The surukuku snake of SouthAmerica N.O. Ophidia.
Trituration. Dilution.

Pathogenetic sphere of action
- The nervous system. causing, cerebral excitation followed by depression.
- Sensory- hyperaesthesia.
- Neuro-vegetative-vaso motor disorders.
- The blood causing haemorrhages. bruises, purpura and congestive blue-violet
  cyanosed condition of skin and mucosa.

Suspicious: fears medicine is a poison.

Jealousy without any reason.

Much loquacity; gives a rambling account of her ailments.

Religious insanity; think she is under super human control.

Oversensitiveness; obliged to wear the clothes very loose especially about
neck, waist etc.

Sun-headache; weight and pressure on vertex; better by onset of discharges.

Vertigo on waking, on closing eyes.

Throat sore, especially left side, worse swallowing liquids, hot drinks.

Throat sensitive to touch, even of linen.

Complaints during climactric period, better by onset of discharges.

Dry cough by pressure on larynx.

Skin bluish, purplish; Bed sores. Senile erysipelas.

Vericose ulcers.

General aggravation in spring season.

Aggravation on entering sleep.

Relieved by discharges, warm applications.

Modalities: Worse after sleep. Lachesis sleeps into aggravation ailments that come on
during sleep. left side. in spring, warm bath. pressure or constriction. hot drinks,
closing eyes. Better appearance of dicharges, warm applications.

Dosage : 200th in fractional dose.

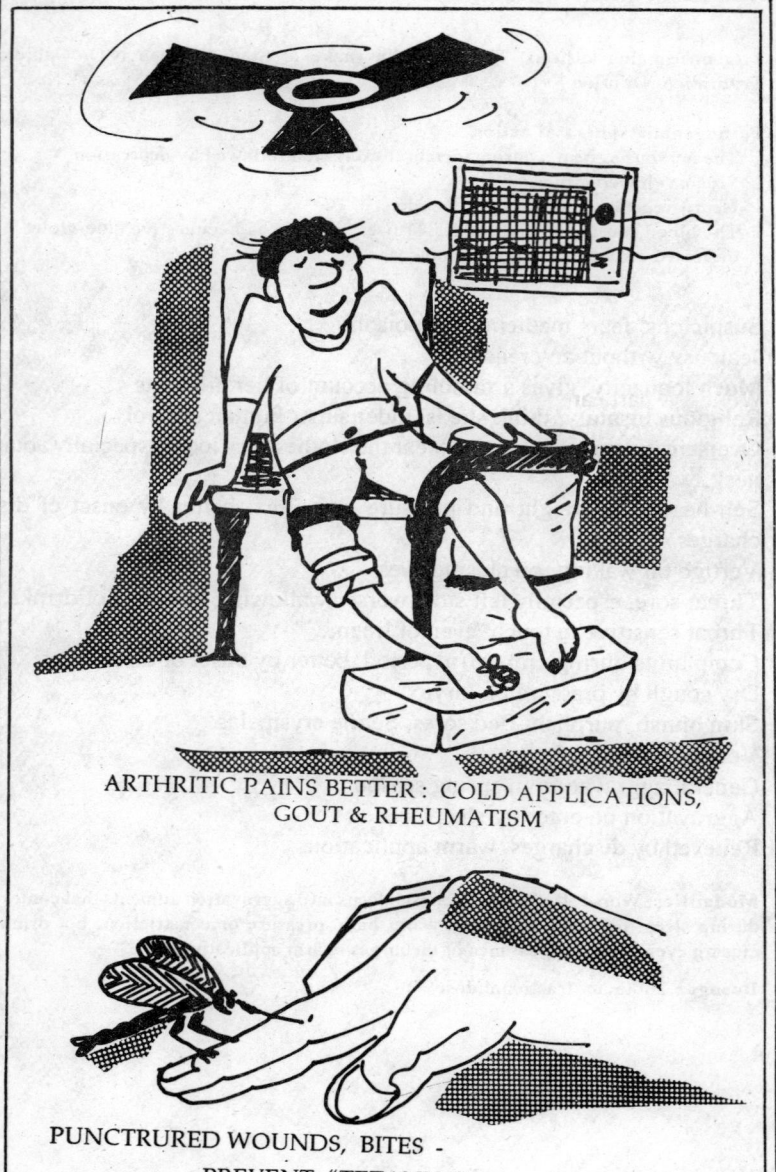

ARTHRITIC PAINS BETTER : COLD APPLICATIONS,
GOUT & RHEUMATISM

PUNCTRURED WOUNDS, BITES -
PREVENT "TETANUS".

LEDUM PALUSTRE

Common name Wild Rosemary. Marsh Cistus. Marsh Tea. Labrador tea. N.O. Ericaceae. Tincture of dried small twigs and leaves collected after flowering begins. Tincture of whole fresh plant.

Pathogenetic sphere of action
- The capillaries causing effusion of blood with dark violet ecchymoses.
- The joints.
- The skin.
- Uric acid metabolism.

General lack of vital heat.

General coldness and yet heat of bed intolerable.

Wounded parts are cold.

Tetanus; prevents tetanus.

Vertigo when walking.

Contusions around eyes. Cataract in gouty subjects.

Red pimples on forehead and cheeks. Acne.

Anal fissures.

Rheumatism and gout, go from below upwards. Stiffness of joints, better applying cold water.

Pains worse from motion, from warmth of bed, at night, better from cold applications. Osteoarthritis.

Patient always sits with the joint exposed to the cold.

It counteracts the bad effects of whisky and takes away the desire for whisky.

Emaciation of affected part.

Punctured wounds, from sharp instruments.

Bites of animals and insect stings.

Ecchymosis. Leucoderma (Vitiligo).

Bluish discolouration after injuries.

Eruptions only on covered parts.

Modalities: Better from cold, putting feet in cold water. Worse at night and from heat of bed.
Dosage: 200th potency 2-3 times (for Anti tetanus action 3 times for 3 days).

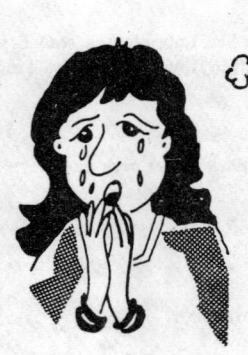
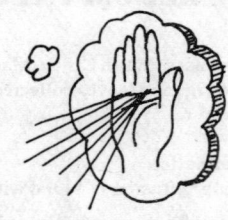

DESPAIR OF SALVATION -

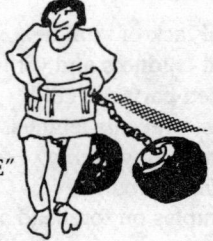

BEARING DOWN PAINS " PROLAPSE"

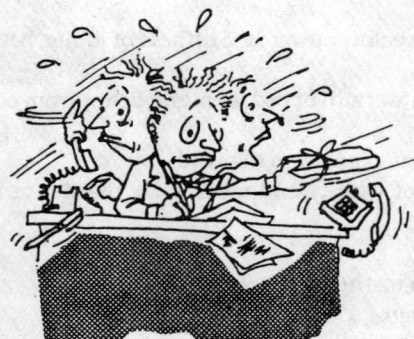

ALWAYS IN HURRY

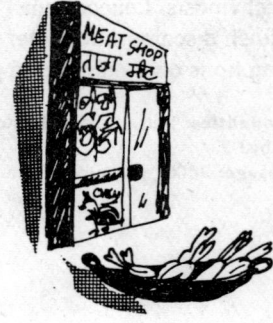

CRAVES MEAT

LILIUM TIGRINUM

Commonly called Tiger Lily. N.O. liliaceae. Tincture of fresh stalk, leaves and flowers.

Pathogenetic sphere of action
- The female genital organs
- The nervous system causing depression and reflex disorders in heart.

Depression of spirits; weeping mood. Consolation aggravates.
Tormented about her salvation.
Uterine complaints.
Constant hurried feeling, as if having too much work to perform and is unable to perform them.
Makes mistakes in writing, in speaking, cannot apply the mind steadily.
Fear of some incurable or fatal disease.
Great craving for meat; ravenous hunger.
Increased thirst.
Aversion to coffee and bread.
Prolapsus uteri.
Bearing down, with sensation of heavy weight and pressure in the region of uterus, as if whole contents would press out through vagina.
Has to support by upward pressure of the hand.
Retroversion of uterus.
Continual pressure in bladder, wants to urinate all the time.
Continual pressure on rectum and anus with a contant desire to go to stool.
Sharp pains in ovarian region. Ovary swollen.
Heart were grasped or squeezed in a vice.
Constrictive pain in heart. Much palpitatoin.
Complaints following miscarriage and sub-involution of uterus.

Modalities: Worse consolation, warm room. Better fresh air.

Dosage : 200th or higher, one dose and wait.

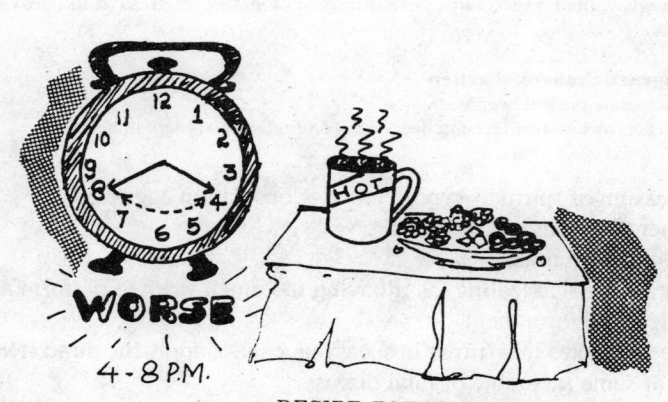

WORSE

4 - 8 P.M.

DESIRE FOR HOT, SWEETS.

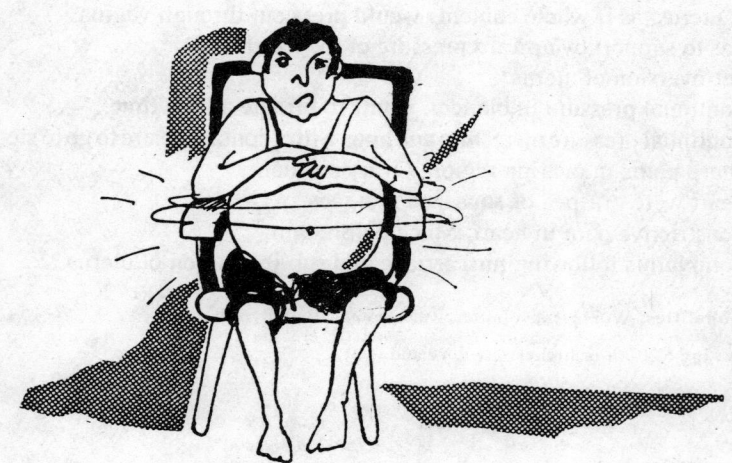

EXCESSIVE DISTENSION BY FLATULENCE,
HYPERACIDITY OR ASCITES.

LYCOPODIUM CLAVATUM

Commonly called lycopodium Clavatum. Common name - Club moss. Wolf's - claw. N.O. lycopodiaceae.Trituration of spores.

Pathogenetic sphere of action
- The liver and digestive function.
- The kidneys and genital system.
- The mucosa and skin.
- The nervous system causing asthenia both physical and psychic.

Aversion to company, and yet he dreads solitude.
Sensitive - even cries when thanked; at the slightest joy.
Speaks wrong words and syllables.
Select wrong words.
Absent minded; thinks he is in two places at the same time.
Despondent.
Want of self confidence, indecision, timidity.
Distrustful, suspicious and fault finding.
Headache, worse from heat and better from cold fresh air.
Hair falls and become grey too early.
General aggravation in afternoon, from 4 to 8 p.m.
Desires hot drinks and sweets.
Great acidity and flatulence.Excessive bloating of abdomen.
Liver enlarged and painful. Ascitis from liver diseases.
Gall-stone colic.
Hernia - right sided.
Haemorrhoides, painful, bleeding.
Right sided renal calculi.
Dyspnoea, night cough.
Sleepy during the day, wakeful at night.

Modalities: Worse right side, from right to left, form above downward, 4-8 p.m. from heat or warm room, hot air, bed, warm applications, except throat and stomach which are better from warm drinks. Better by motion, after midnight, from warm food and drink, on getting cold, from being uncovered.

Dosage : 200th or higher infrequently 200th frequently in colics.

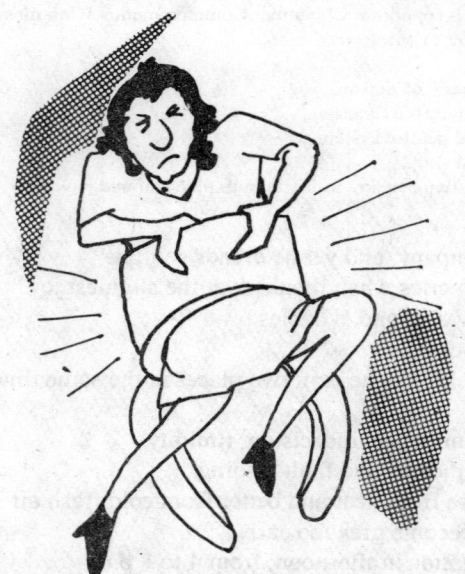

SPASMS, CRAMPS AND COLICS

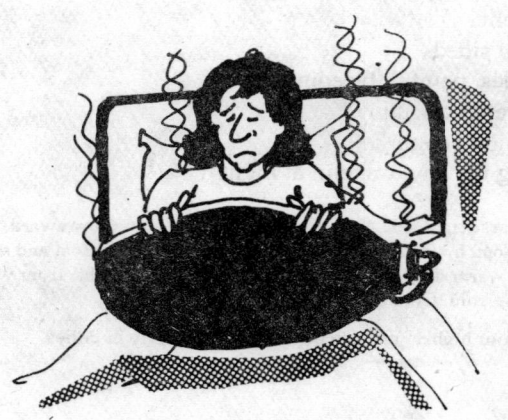

BETTER: WARM APPLICATIONS

MAGNESIA PHOSPHORICA

Phosphate of Magnesia (MgHPO$_4$,H$_2$O) Trituration.

Pathogenetic sphere of action. It has a major action on spasms.

It has a major action on spasms.

Spasms, cramps, neuralgic pains, and colics all relieved by heat and pressure.

Neuralgias, especially on right side and of face.

Trigeminal neuralgia.

Toothache, better by heat and hot liquids.

Rheumatic headaches; better by external warmth.

Strabismus and Nystagmus.

Complaints of teething children.

Violent abdominal colic, forcing the patient to bend double; relieved by pressure and warm application.

Membranous dysmenorrhoea.

Whooping cough; spasmodic cough.

Angina-pectoris with nervous palpitation.

Convulsions with stiffness of the limbs.

Sciatica right sided; shooting pain along with the nerves.

Chorea, writer's and player's cramps.

Nocturnal enuresis from nervous irritation.

Chilliness; chill run up and down the back with shivering.

Modalities: Worse right side, cold, touch, night Better warmth, bending double, pressure friction.

Dosage : 6x in hot water in colics. 200th or higher in neuralgias.

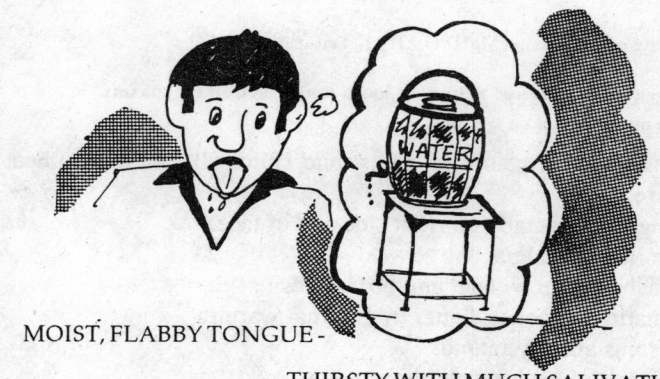

MOIST, FLABBY TONGUE -

THIRSTY WITH MUCH SALIVATION

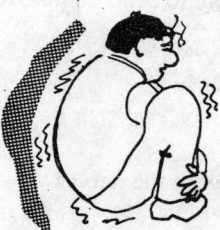

- CHILLY

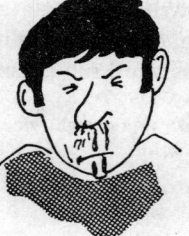

NOSE DIRTY (ALWAYS CLOGGED WITH
THICK GREEN DISCHARGE)

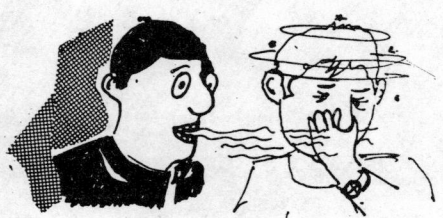

FETID DISCHARGES

MERCURIUS SOLUBILIS

Mercurius solubilis Hahnemanni. Dimercuros ammonium Nitrate $2(NH_2Hg_2)$ $NO3H_2O$.
Trituration.

Pathogenetic sphere of action
- The digestive mucosa, from mouth to rectum
- The genito urinary mucosa and renal parenchyma.
- The skin causing inflammation with tendency towards suppuration.

Hurried and rapid talking.
Weak memory; forgets easily. Slow in answering questions.
Homesickness.
Whole head is painful to touch.
Itching on the scalp, loss of hair.
Vertigo when lying on back.
Great sliminess of mucous membranes.
Otaligia-yellow, thick discharge; worse warmth of bed.
Nostrils raw, ulcerated with green, fetid discharge.
Excessive salivation; saliva tastes metallic or sweetish or fetid. Gums
spongy, bleeding.
Crown of teeth decayed. Teeth loose, tender.
Tongue moist, thick, flabby, with imprints of teeth.
Ulceration and inflammation of throat.
Intense thirst for cold drinks with increased hunger.
Dysentery-bloody, slimy stool, worse at night; and great tenesmus.
Cannot lie on right side.
Worse from the heat of bed, at night.
Profuse perspiration.
Sensitive to heat and cold.
Bone pains, worse at night.
Glands are inflamed and swollen. Tendency to ulcerate.
Ulcers sting and burns, with lardaceous base.

Modalities: Worse at night, wet damp weather, lying on right side, perspiring, warm
room and warm bed.

Dosage : 30th in abdominal complaints, 200th in all oral complaints.

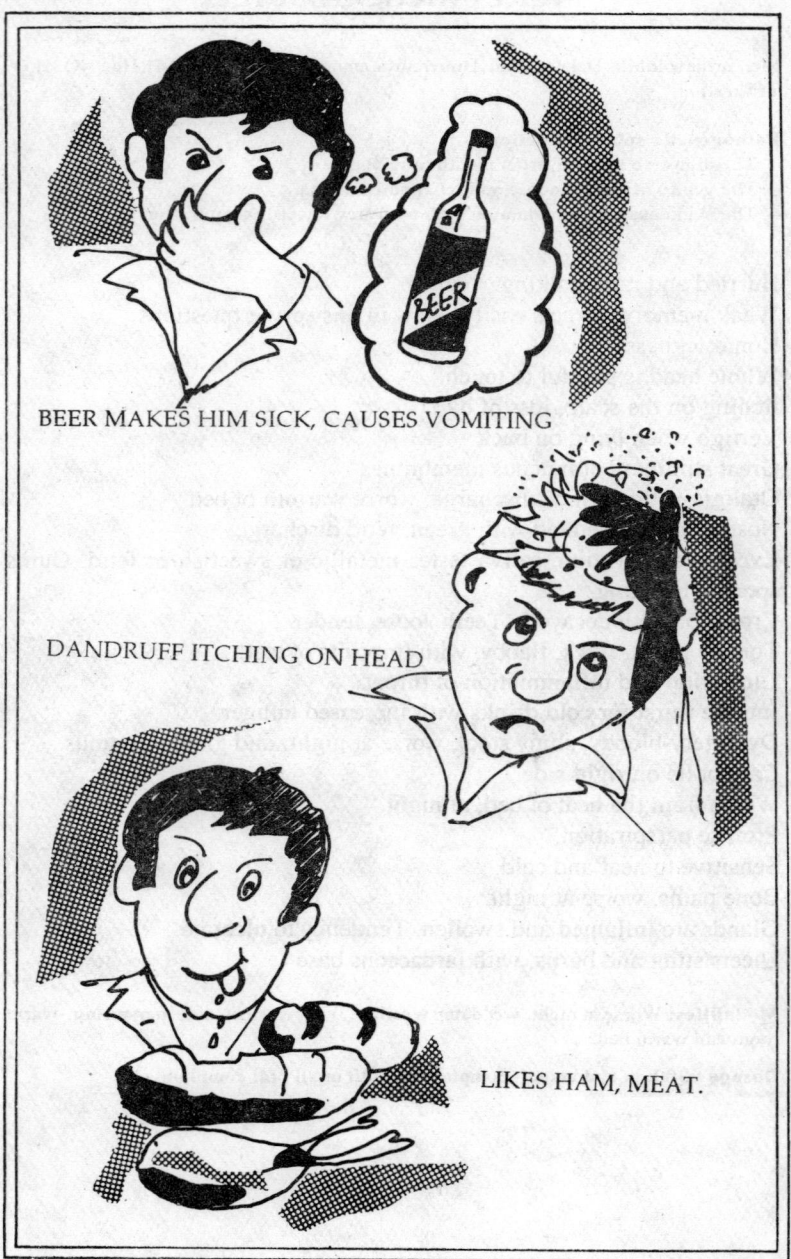

BEER MAKES HIM SICK, CAUSES VOMITING

DANDRUFF ITCHING ON HEAD

LIKES HAM, MEAT.

MEZEREUM

Daphne mezereum. spurge olive. N.O. Thymelaceae. Tincture of fresh bark gathered just before the plant flowers in february and March.

Pathogenetic sphere of action
- The mucosa and periosteum causing irritation particularly in the malar region.
- The skin causing irritation with purulent and vesiculo-scabby eruptions.

Hypochondriac and despondent.

Great chilliness and sensitiveness to cold air.

Marked action on skin, bones and mucous membranes.

Stupefying headache on right side.

Scalp covered with thick, leather crusts, under which pus collects.

Dandruff.

Deafness, ears feels wide open as though cold air were blowing in.

Ciliary neuralgia after eye operation.

Red eruptions around mouth.

Desires for ham, meat.

Excessive salivation. Beer causes vomiting.

Chronic gastritis. Gastic Ulcer.

Enlargement of testicles. Gonorrhoea with haematuria.

Pain in neck and back, worse, motions and at night.

Violent pains in long bones, esp. at night and in damp weather. Caries of bones. Exostosis. Eczema, intolerable itching.

Eruptions ulcerate and form thick scabs under which pus exudes.

Localised twitching of small groups of muscles.

Modalities: Worse cold air, night, evening until midnight, warm food, touch, motion. Better open air.

Dosage : 30th twice daily in eczema.Higher in neuralgias.

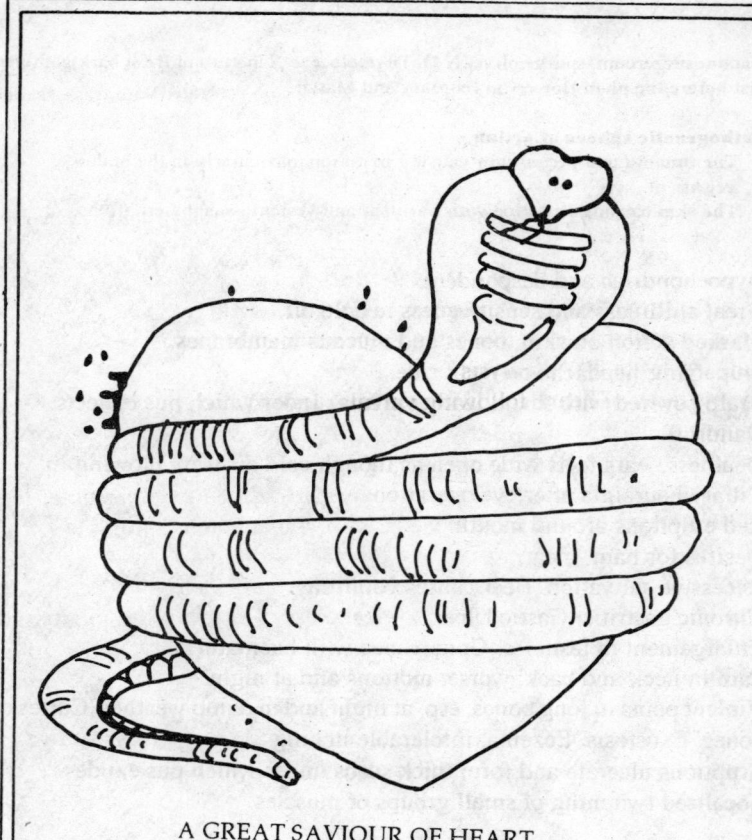

A GREAT SAVIOUR OF HEART

NAJA

Commonly called Naja tripudians. The hooked snake of Hindustan. N.O.Elapidae.
Tincture of the fresh venom.Trituration of sugar of milk saturated with fresh venom.

Pathogenetic sphere of action
- The nervous system
- The blood
- It has predominant effect upon the nerves of the heart causing palpitations and precordial pain.

Its action settles around the heart.

Heart; valvular lesions following rheumatic fever.

Naja causes bulbar paralysis.

Hypertrophy of heart, following valvular lesion.

Organs seem to be drawn together.

Very susceptible to cold.

Headache; forehead and temples with heart ailments; left temple, left orbital region, extending to occiput, with nausea and vomiting.

Irritating dry cough, dependant on cardiac lesion.

Asthma; begining with coryza.

Angina; extending to nape of neck, left shoulder, left arm with anxiety and fear of death.

Pulse irregular.

Acute and chronic endocarditis.

Left ovarian neuralgia; seems to be drawn to heart.

Sleep, as if raptile is sleeping; deep.

A GREAT SAVIOUR OF HEART.

Modalities: Worse from use of stimulants. Better from walking or riding in open air.

Dosage : 30th few doses.

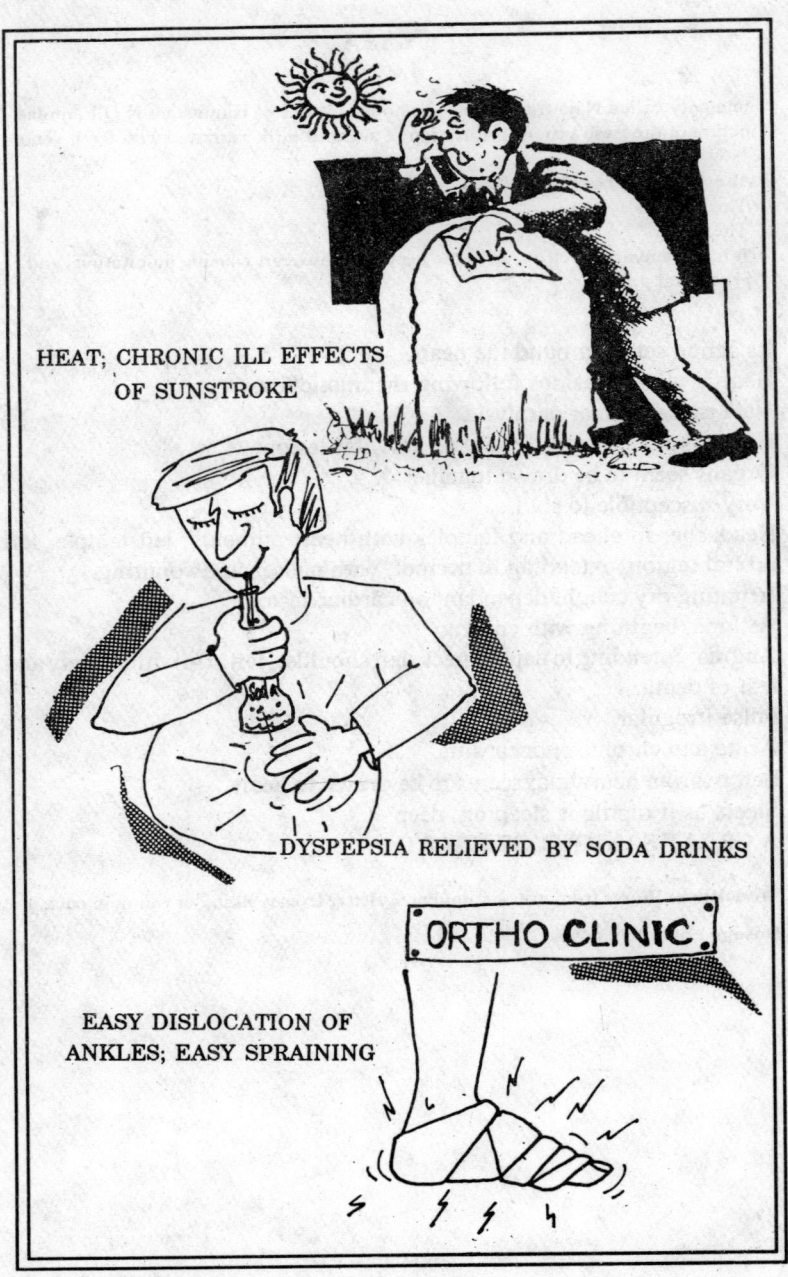

HEAT; CHRONIC ILL EFFECTS
OF SUNSTROKE

DYSPEPSIA RELIEVED BY SODA DRINKS

ORTHO CLINIC

EASY DISLOCATION OF
ANKLES; EASY SPRAINING

NATRUM CARBONICUM

Sodium Carbonate $Na_2CO_{3\ 10}\ H_2O$. Trituration solution.

Pathogenetic sphere of action
- The nervous system causing depression with sensorial hyperaesthesia particularly of auditory type.
- The digestive mucosa causing irritation.

Great debility caused by summer heat., chronic effect of sunstroke exhaustion, anaemic, milky, watery skin, weak ankles.
Headache from slightest mental exertion worse from sun or working under gas light.
Catarrah bad smell of nasal secretion, posterior nasal catarrah.
Hawking much mucus from throat worse slightest error in diet.
Yellow substance like pulp of orange in stools.
Easy dislocation and spraining of ankles.
Dyspepsia better by soda drinks.

Modalities: Worse sitting, music, summer heat, mental exertion, thunder storm, least draught, changes of weather, sun. Better by moving, by boring in ears, and nose.

Dosage : 30th few doses a day.

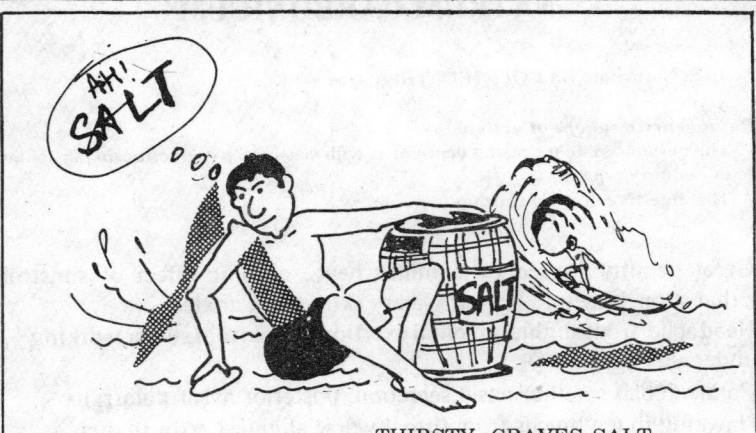

THIRSTY, CRAVES SALT

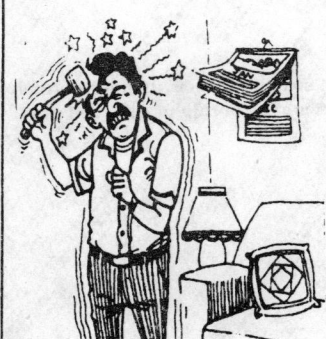

HAMMERING HEADACHE
"ANAEMIC HEADACHE"

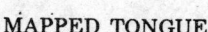
MAPPED TONGUE.

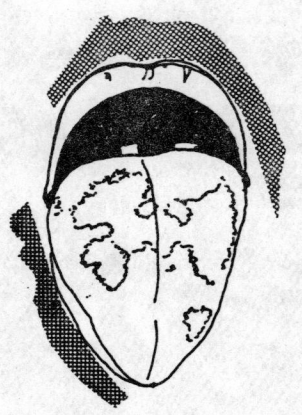

NATRUM MURIATICUM

Sodium Chloride. Common salt. NaCl. Trituration. Solution.

Pathogenetic sphere of action
- Nutrition- causing disassimilation.
- The kidney.
- The stomach
- The blood causing anaemia.
- The mucosa, causing dryness or a secondary catarrhal condition characterized by excessive secretion of mucus.
- The skin-causing increase of flow of sebum particularly on face and forehead.
- The nervous system-causing depressive syndrome.

Hates sympathy, fuss and company.

Craves salt.

Lothes fat.

Worse at sea side.

Depressed; weeping tendency, consolation aggravates.

Bad effects of grief, fright, anger etc.

Headache, from sunshine to sunset.

Chronic anaemic headache of school girls.

Hammering headache.

Eye muscles weak and stiff. Lachrymation.

Violent fluent coryza with discharge like raw white of an egg.

Violent sneezing.

Loss of smell and taste.

Sensation of hair on tongue. Tongue mapped.

Deep fissured crack in the centre of lower lip.

Sweat while eating. Aversion to bread. Increased thirst.

Involuntary urination on coughing and sneezing etc.

Cannot pass urine if others are present.

Pain in back, with desire for some firm support.

Numbness and tingling in fingers etc.

Palms hot and perspiring.

Skin oily. Dry crusts on margin of hairy scalp and bends of joints.

Warts on palms of hands.

General aggravation about 11 a.m.

Coldness of body and continued chilliness.

Modalities: Worse noise, music, warm room, lying down, about 10 a.m. at seashore, mental exertion, consolation, heat, talking. Better open air, cold bathing, going without regular meals lying on right side, pressure against back, tight clothing.

Dosage : 30th in acute complaints,200th or higher when used constitutionally.

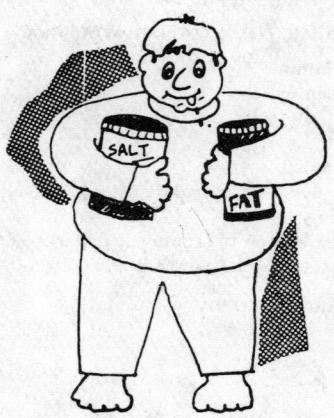

LIKING FOR FATS AND SALT

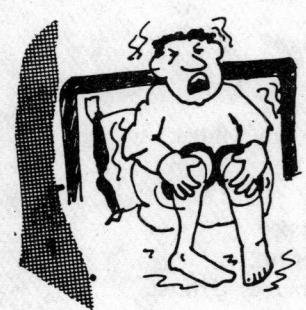

CHILLY - LIMBS ACHING

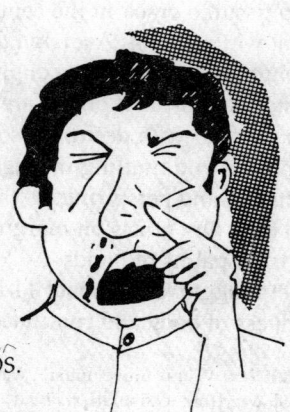

ITCHING IN NOSE NOSE BLEEDS.

NITRIC ACID

Nitric Acid, Aquafortis HNO$_3$, Solution.

Pathogenetic sphere of action
- The mucosa particularly in the cutaneous mucous junction.

Chilly; depressed; indifferent.
Intolerance of sympathy.
Sensitive to noise, pain, touch, jar.
Irritable; suspicious; obstinate; restless.
Fear of death.
Great weakness of memory.
Likes fat, salt.
Headache - sensation as if head is in a vice from ear to ear, over vertex.
Vertigo in morning.
Profuse falling of hair.
Double vision.
Roaring in ears; deafness.
Violent itching in nose. Nose bleeds.
Corners of mouth ulcerated and scabby with foul smell form mouth.
Bloody saliva.
Ulcers in soft palate, with sharp splinter like pain.
Craves indigestible things.
Fissure in rectum, violent pains after stools.
Prolapsus ani. Haemorrhoids which bleeds easily.
Urine-offensive, smell like horse's urine.
Haemoptysis. Fetid foot sweats.
Wart, large, jagged, bleed on washing.
Ulcers bleed easily. Sensitive; splinter like pain. Irregular edges of ulcers, base of ulcer looks like raw flesh.
Haemorrhages, bright and profuse.

Modalities: Worse evening and night, cold climate and hot weather. Better while riding in carriage.

Dosage : 200th one or two doses daily.

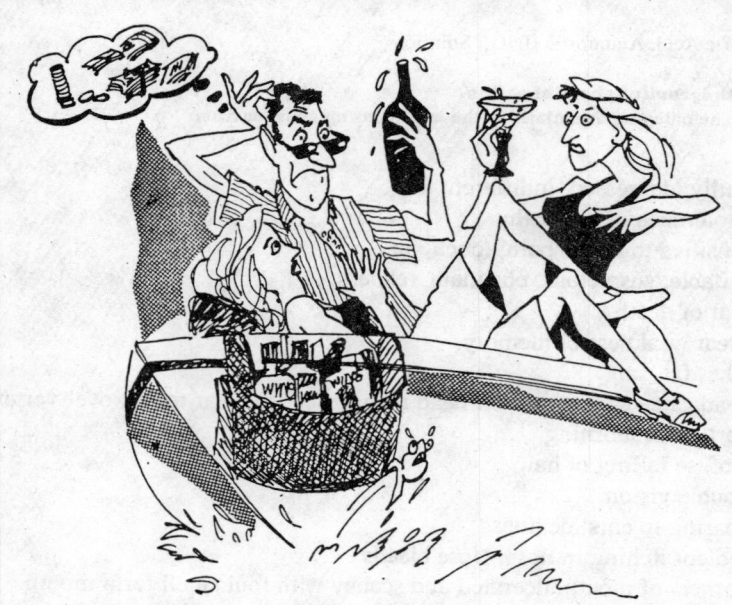

EXTREMELY IRRITABLE, ARISTOCRAT, HIGH LIVING

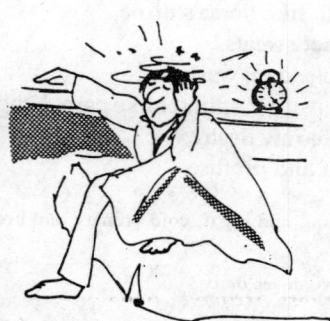

HEADACHE & GIDDINESS IN MORNING "THE MODERN MAN"

NUX VOMICA

Strychnos nux vomica. Common name Poison nut. N.O. loganiaceae. Tincture and trituration of imported seeds.

Pathogenetic sphere of action
- The nervous system
- The digestive tract

Irritable, nervous, zealous, fiery temperament.

Oversensitive to impressions.

Quarrelsome, fault finding.

Sensitive to noises, odours, light etc.

Indulges in too much mental work, lives sedentary life, takes rich and stimulating food, and drinks tea, coffee, wine etc. possibly in excess.

Hypochondriasis due to digestive disturbances and congestion.

Extremely chilly, worse in open air.

Headache in morning; in sunshine with giddiness.

Stuffy cold after exposure to cold. Coryza fluent in day and dry at night.

Painful, tickling sore throat.

Nausea in morning, after breakfast. Weight and pain in stomach, especially following some time after eating.

Heartburn, water brash.

Loves fats and tolerates them well.

Dyspepsia of tea and coffee drinkers.

Liver enlarged and painful, especially in alcoholics.

Constipation, with ineffecutal desire, feels as if some part remained unexpelled.

Haemorrhoids, itching, painful, do not bleed.

Dysentery; stools relieve pains for some time.

Asthma with fullness in stomach; worse in morning or after eating.

Cough causes bursting headache.

Backache in lumbar region. Must sit up in order to turn in bed; worse 3-4 a.m.

Cannot sleep after 3 a.m. till morning; sleepy in morning.

Spastic, jerking of limbs and feeling of wearines in limbs.

Partial paralysis.

Body burning hot; yet cannot uncover, as feels too much chilly.

Suits thin, mental workers, irritable, wine, wealth and women play an important role in their lives.

Modalities: Worse morning, mental exertion, after eating, touch, spices, stimulants, narcotis, dry weather, cold. Better from a nap, if allowed to finish it, in evening, while at rest, in damp, wet weather, strong pressure.

Dosage : 30th 3 times daily for some time (as it takes time to show action).

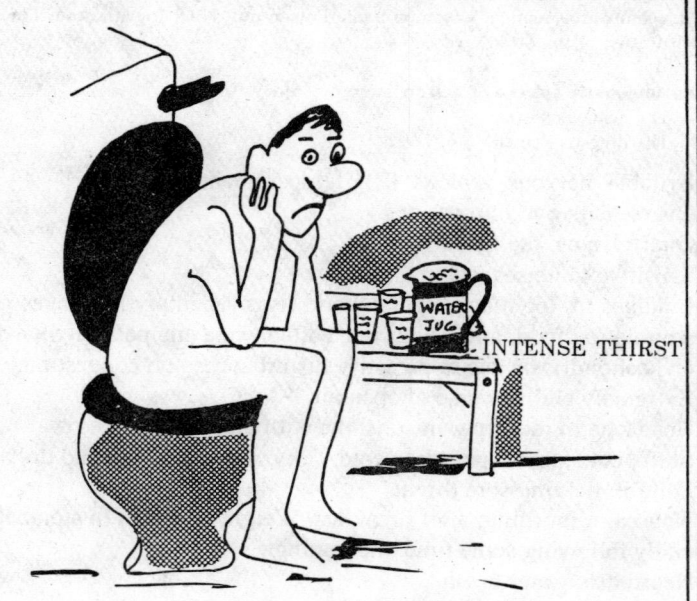

INTENSE THIRST

PAINLESSNESS CONSTIPATION

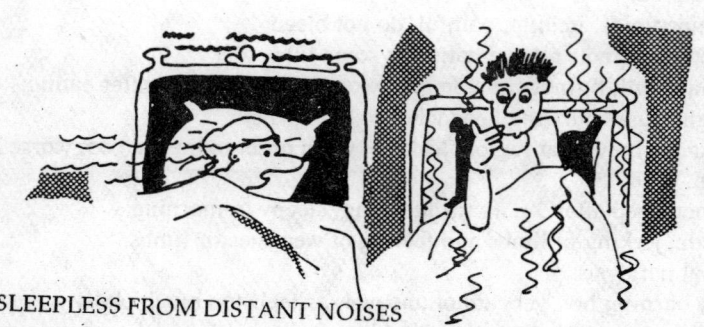

SLEEPLESS FROM DISTANT NOISES

LIMBS TWITCH, BED FEELS HOT.

OPIUM

Papaver somniferum. Poppy. N.O. Papaveraceae. Tincture.

Pathogenetic sphere of action
- An initial phase of cerebral hyperactivity with euphoria and auditory hypersenstivity.
- There is second phase of slowing down with prostration, lack of sensitivity and indolence.
- There is intestinal paresis with decrease of all secretions except for perspiration.

Habitual liar, have no conscience left.

No pain. No complaints. No desires.

Complaints from heat, the fright of the fear remains.

Sees frightful images, fire, ghosts, devils etc.

Hears distant voices which prevent sleep.

Eyes glassy, staring, pupils insensible, contracted.

Tongue black. Paralyzed.

Intense thirst.

Paralysis.

Fetid vomiting. Strangulated hernia; lead colic.

No desire to eat.

Obstinate constipation, no desire to go to stools for days together; stool, hard, black balls. Faeces protrude and urine retained or involuntary.

Deep, stertorous breathing, deep snoring.

Sleep - heavy, deep, profound coma. Feels bed is hot, much sweating.

Twitching of limbs; numbness.

Convulsions, worse from light.

Hot sweat over whole body except lower limbs.

Marasums; child wrinkled and looks like a little dried up old man.

Modalities: Worse heat, during and after sleep. Better cold things, constant walking.

Dosage : 30th for constipation. Highear infrequent doses for neurological deficits.

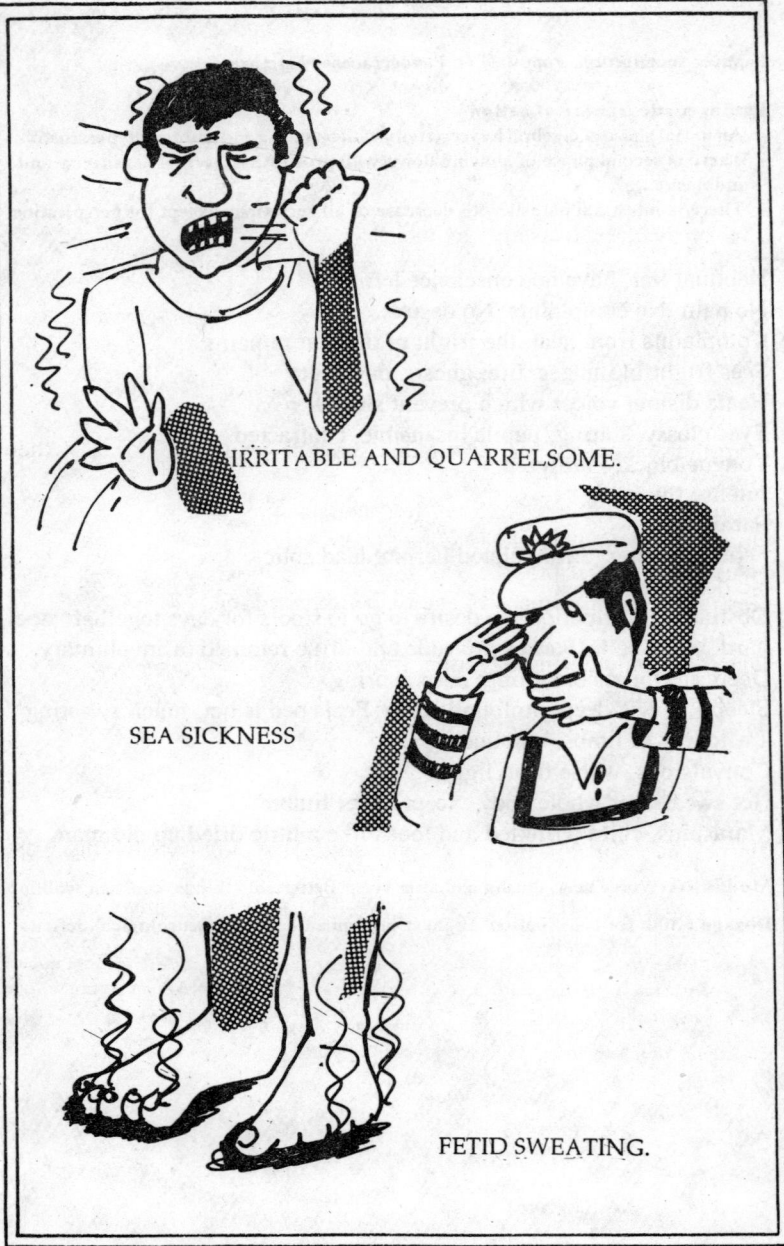

IRRITABLE AND QUARRELSOME.

SEA SICKNESS

FETID SWEATING.

PETROLEUM

Oleum petrae. Rock oil, Coal oil. Trituration and tincture of the rectified oil.

Pathogenetic sphere of action
- The skin causing irritation with first vesicular then scab like eruptions.
- The digestive mucosa causing catarrhal irritation with hunger after each stool.

Low spirited, quarrelsome; irritable.
Feels that death is near and must hurry to settle affairs.
Thinks he is double.
Occiput heavy, as of lead.
Headache from cold breeze.
SEA SICKNESS. Vertigo on rising.
Moist eruptions on scalp.
Marginal blepharitis. Dim sighted, cannot read fine prints without glasses.
Nostrils cracked, ulcerated, burn, Epistaxis.
Hunger, immediately after stools.
Nausea with water brash.
Gastralgia when stomach is empty; better by eating.
Ravenous hunger.
Diarrhoea only during day time; from eating cabbage.
Itching of anus.
Tips of fingers cracked, rough, fissured every winter.
Crackling in joints; worse in winter.
Skin rough scaly, leathery.
Rhagades, worse in winter.
Herpes; eczema with thick, greenish crusts, burning and itching; worse in winter.
Fetid sweat in axillae, between thighs and under breasts.

Modalities: Worse dampness, before and during a thunderstorm, from riding in cars, passive motion, in winter, eating, from mental staress. Better warm air, lying with head high, dry weather.

Dosage : 30th few doses daily. 200th before journey.

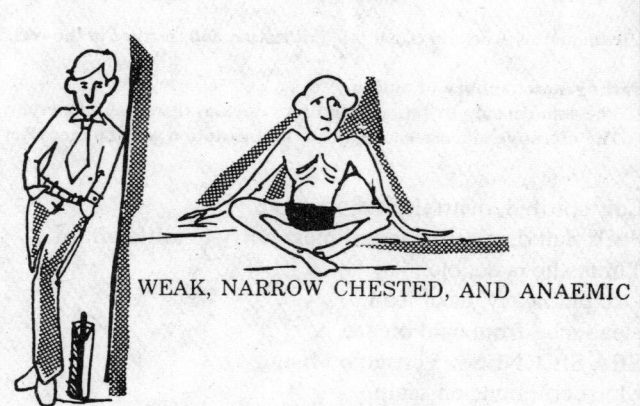

WEAK, NARROW CHESTED, AND ANAEMIC

THIN, TALL, PERSONS : RELIEVED BY SHORT SLEEP

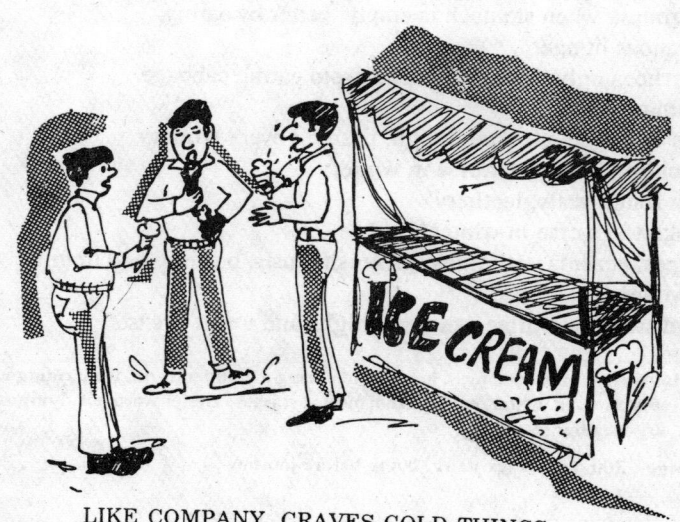

LIKE COMPANY, CRAVES COLD THINGS

PHOSPHORUS

The element   Saturated solution in absolute alochol.Trituration of red amorphous phosphorus.

Pathogenetic sphere of action
- All the parenchymatous tissues particularly of the hepatic, pulmonary and renal parenchyma, causing intense congestion with haemorrhage and fatty degeneration.

Lean, thin, narrow chested, tubercular type of patient.
Fine, soft hair, delicate personality.
Great susceptibility to external impressions, like light, sounds, thunder stroms etc.
Great lowness of spirits.
Great apathy; indifferent to friends etc.
Fear something will happen; anxious at twilight.
Fear of strange, insane imaginations.
Like company. Fear of death; worse when alone.
Vertigo after rising. Heat comes from occiput.
Dandruff; falling of hair in bunches.
Photophobia; letter appear red.
Atrophy of optic nerve; thrombosis of retinal vessels.
Sensation of fog or mist before eyes.
Epistaxis; bright red blood. Nasal polypi.
Thirst for very cold, icy drinks.
Craving for salt. Ice cream.
Vomiting of water as soon as it gets warm.
Painless, debilitating diarrhoea, very offensive flatus.
Larynx very painful. Cannot talk on account of pain.
Cough; worse talking, cold air, laughing etc.
Tightness across the chest; breathing quickened, oppressed; worse lying on left side.
Haemoptysis. Post diphtheric paralysis.
Sleep short with frequent waking.
Haemorrhagic tendency, scurvy. Purpura haemorrhagica.

Modalities: Worse, touch, physical or mental exertion, twilight, warm food or drink, change of weather, from getting wet in hot weather, evening, lying on left or painful side during a thunderstorm, ascending stairs. Better in dark, lying on right side, cold, food, cold, open air, washing with cold water, sleep.

Dosage : 30th or 200th few doses and wait for action.

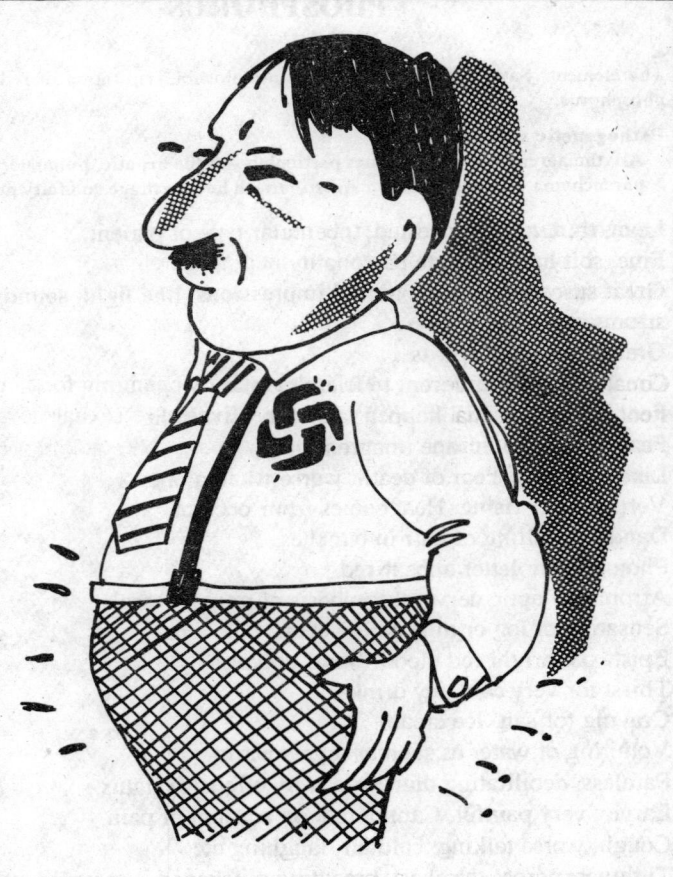

ARROGANT
FALSE SELF-ADMIRATION AND CONTEMPT FOR OTHERS

PLATINA

Platinum. An element.Pt. (A.W. 194.3) Trituration.

Pathogenetic sphere of action
- The nervous system
- The female genital system.

Arrogant, proud, contempt for others.
Physical symptoms alternates with mental symptoms.
Headache; cramping. squeezing with numbness. Objects look smaller than they are. Painter's colic, pain in umblical region, extending through to back.
Constipation of travellers who are constantly changing food, and water; stool sticky, evacuated with difficulty. Excessive sexual development, parts sensitive; menses too early, too profuse, dark, clotted.
Sterility with nymphomania; sleep with legs apart.

Modalities: Worse sitting and standing, evening. Better walking.

Dosage : 200th or higher few doses.

132

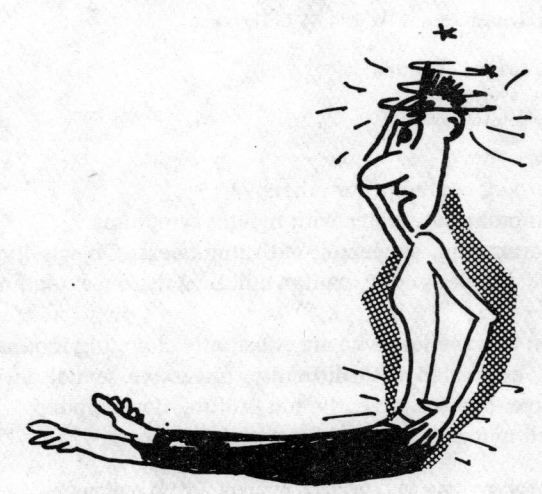

AS IF ABDOMEN WERE DRAWN TO SPINE BY A STRING
"COLIC WITH RETRACTED ABDOMEN"

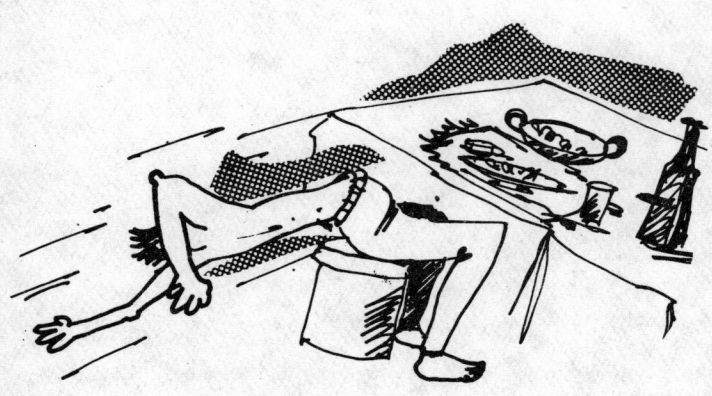

FAINTNESS AND PROSTRATION AFTER MEALS.

PLUMBUM METALLICUM

Plumbum Metallicum. The element Pb(A.W.206.39). Trituration.

Pathogenetic sphere of action
- The digestive system
- The circulatory system causing arterial vasoconstriction with secondary arterio-sclerosis and renal damage.
- The nervous sytem causing progressive paresis, paralysis and muscular atrophy.

Mental depression; slowness of perception. Loss of memory.
Fear of being assassinated. Paretic weakness.
Headache; anaemia and emaciation with general prostration.
Tinnitus.
Glaucoma.
Dark blue line on the gums. Breath fetid.
Loss of appetite. Nausea. Vomiting.
Gastralgia; extremely violent pains in the umbelical region.
Retracted abdomen; navel seems to adhere to the spine.
Constipation; stools hard, dry, like sheep's dung, with terrible urging and pain from constriction and spasm of anus.
Bright's disease.
Contracted kidney.
Vaginismus, induration of mammary glands. Menorrhagia.
Violent pains in the extremities, especially in evening and night.
Jerking, trembling and numbness of limbs.
Wrist drop. Pain in muscles of thigh, comes in paroxysms.
Progressive muscular atrophy; from sclerosis of spinal cord.
Delirium. Coma; convulsions. Excessive hyperaesthesia or anaesthesia.
Arthralgia. Infantile paralysis.
Lassitude and faintness.
Skin dry and yellow.
Sleeplessness.
Hypertension. Arteriosclerosis.

Modalities: Worse at night, motion. Better rubbing, hard pressure, physical exertion.

Dosage : 30th and higher for paralytic ailments.

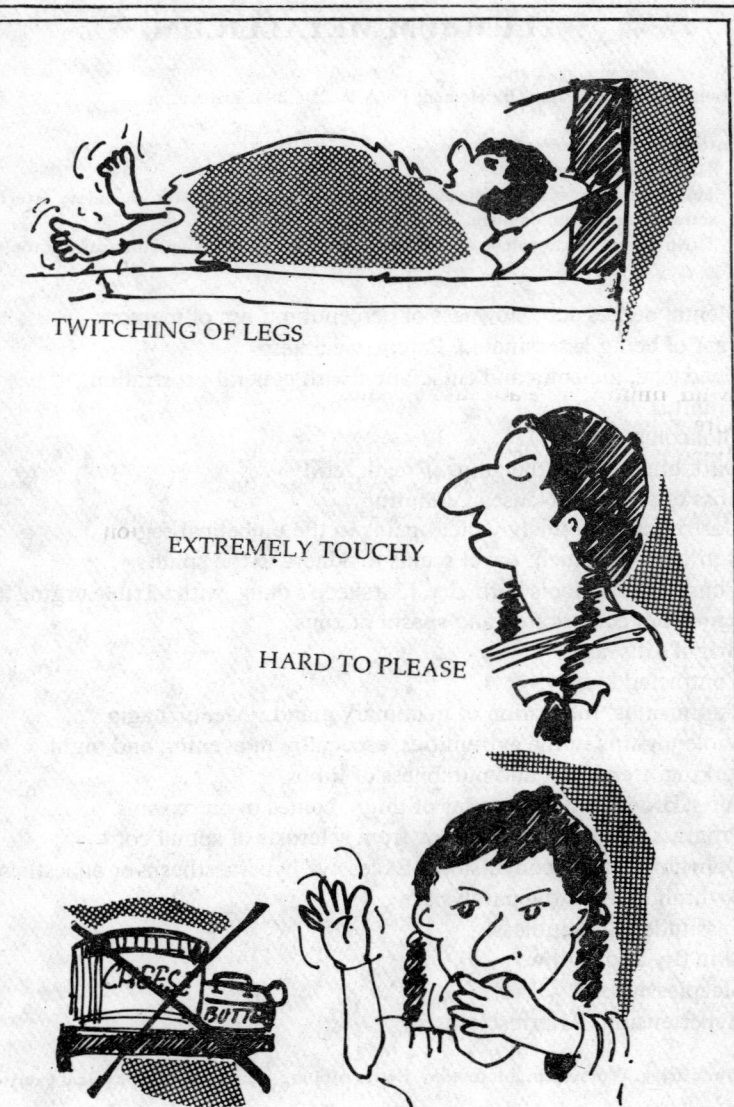

TWITCHING OF LEGS

EXTREMELY TOUCHY

HARD TO PLEASE

DISLIKE CHEESE AND BUTTER.

PULSATILLA NIGRICANS

Anemone pratensis. Common name Pasque flower.N.O.Ranunculaceae. Tincture of entire fresh plant when in flower.

Pathogenetic sphere of action
- The mucosa causing catarrhal state particularly of digestive, respiratory and genital mucosa with yellow or greenish yellow, thick, non irritating discharge.
- The venous system causing congestion and stasis.

No thirst, no hunger.

Weepy; cannot tell her symptoms without tears.

Changeable.

Very responsive to sympathy.

Mild, timid, gentle and affectionate.

Great fear of insanity.

Imaginative; jealous; suspicious. Hard to please.

Vertigo, as if intoxicated, especially when sitting.

Heaviness of head; craves open air; better in open air.

Itching, burning in eyes. Lachrymation.

Tongue coated with viscid mucus.

Aggravation from fats and rich food, butter, pastry, etc.

Thirstlessness.

Taste putrid; nausea and vomiting.

Eructations of food taken long before.

Flatulent colic.

Menses suppressed, delayed or intermittent.

Dry cough in evening or night, loose cough in morning with greenish, profuse, lumpy expectoration.

Drawing, tensive pains in thigh and legs; worse from letting the affected part hang down.

Varicose veins.

Measles.

Urticaria from rich food.

Sleepless in first part of night.

Modalities: Worse from heat, rich fat food, after eating, towards evening, warm room, lying on left or on painless side. when allowing feet to hang down. Better open air, motion. cold application. cold food and drinks, though not thirsty.

Dosage : 30th in acute complaints 200th and higher for functional amenorrhoea.

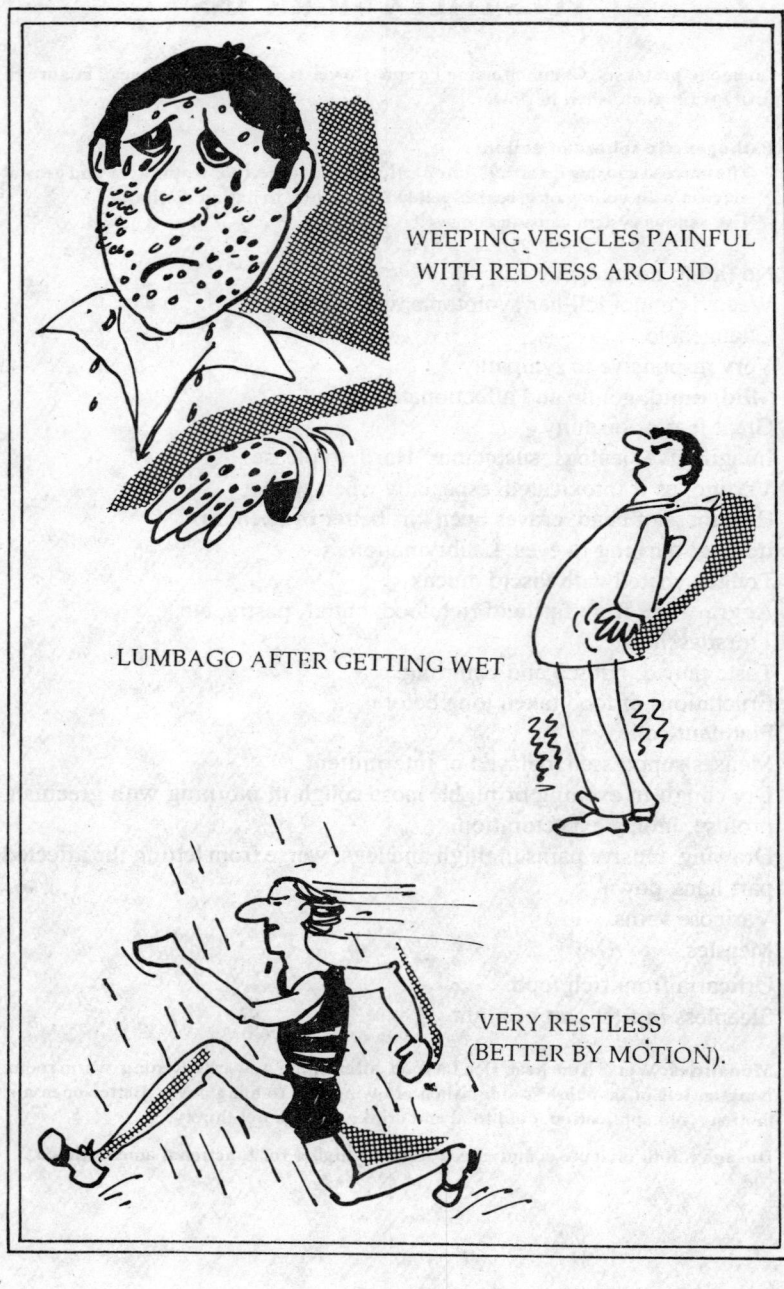

WEEPING VESICLES PAINFUL
WITH REDNESS AROUND

LUMBAGO AFTER GETTING WET

VERY RESTLESS
(BETTER BY MOTION).

RHUS TOXICODENDRON

Common name Poison oak. N.O. Anacar diaceae. Tincture of fresh leaves gathered at sunset just before flowering time.

Pathogenetic sphere of action
- The skin causing oedema and vesicular eruptions.
- The mucosa causing irritation.
- The periarticular fibro connective tissue causing painful stiffness relieved by motion.
- The nervous system causing depression.

Extremely restless, must change position.

Sensorium cloudy, great apprehension at night.

Fear of being poisoned.

Low spirited and inclined to weep.

Scalp sensitive to touch, with humid eruptions on scalp; with great itching.

Orbital cellulitis, pustular eruptions.

Old eye injuries.

Jaws crack when chewing.

Face swollen, facial neuralgia.

Bitter taste in mouth.

Desire for milk. Great thirst.

Swelling and stiffness of joints; lumbago, painful rheumatic affections of joints, muscles and aponeuroses; fibrositis.

All worse form rain and damp weather and when resting; when from movement, though first movement painful.

Burning, tingling, painful vesicular eruptions of skin.

Dilatation of heart in athletes and men who handle heavy tools.

Strained feeling from over exertion.

Paralysis.

Modalities: Worse during sleep, cold, wet rainy weather and after rain, at night, during rest, drenching, when lying on back or right side. Better warm, dry weather, motion, walking, change of position, rubbing, warm applications, from streching limbs.

Dosage : 6th or 30th for acute ailments. 1000 or higher for sprains and strains.

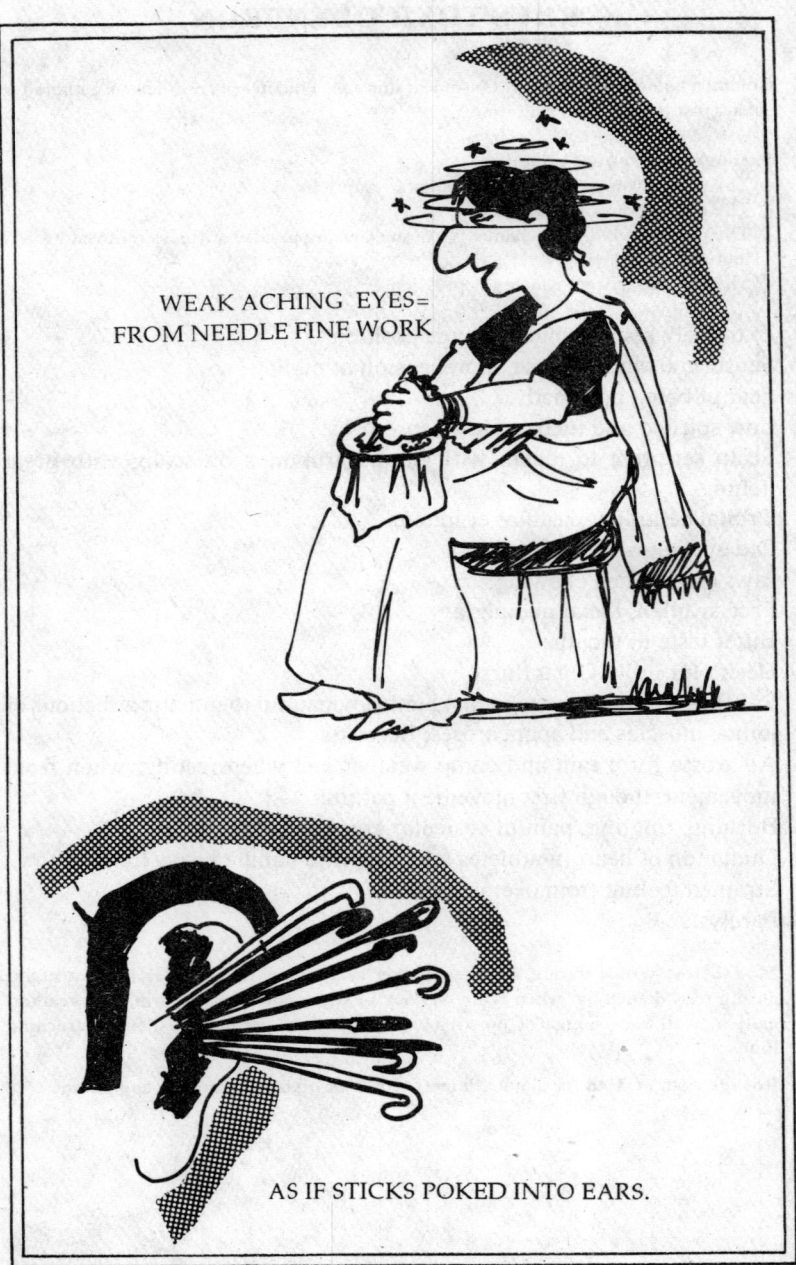

WEAK ACHING EYES=
FROM NEEDLE FINE WORK

AS IF STICKS POKED INTO EARS.

RUTA GRAVEOLENS

Commonly called Ruta graveolens. Rue. N.O. Rutaceae.Tincture of whole fresh plant.

Pathogenetic sphere of action
- The fibrous tissue.
- The aponeurosis, tendons and the periosteum.

Feeling of intense lassitude, weakness and despair.
Best action on periosteum, cartilages, eyes and uterus.
Eye strain follwed by headache.
Eyes red, hot and painful from sewing or reading fine prints.
Distrubance of accomodation.
Overstrained ocular muscles.
Pressure over eye brows. Asthenopia.
Feeling as if blunt sticks were being poked in ears.
Difficult faces, constipation.
Carcinoma affecting lower bowel.
Prolapsus ani every time the bowels move.
Prolplus uteri and ani after confinement.
Lumbago, stiff back.
Spine and limbs bruised.
Deposits in periosteum, tendons and about joints, especially wrist.
Ganglia.
Contraction of fingers.
Sciatica; worse lying down at night.
Tendons sore. Thigh pains when stretching the limbs.
Complaints from straining flexor tendons.
Sprains; injured bruised bones, fractures.
All parts of body on which he lies, even in bed, are painful as if bruised.

Modalities: Worse lying down, from cold, wet weather.

Dosage : 30th for eye and muscular strains.

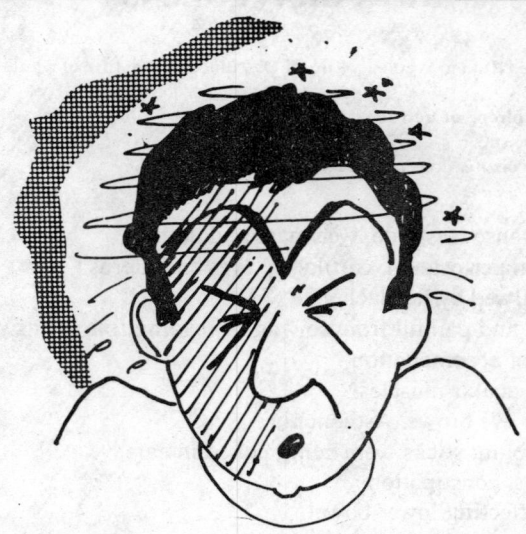

RT. SIDED HEADACHE (SINUSITIS, MIGRAINE OR GASTRIC)

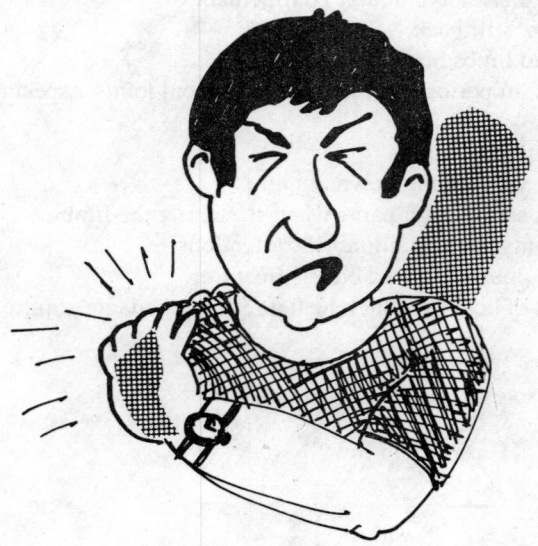

RHEUMATISM: RIGHT SHOULDER.

SANGUINARIA CANADENSIS

Common name blood root. N.O. Papaveraceae. Tincture of fresh root.

Pathogenetic sphere of action
- The circulatory system causing vasomotive disorders, hot flushes, rushing of blood to head with redness confined to cheeks.
- The mucosa causing extreme dryness and there is formationof polyrs which tend to bleed easily.

Periodical sick headache begins in morning, increases during the day, lasts until evening.
Headache begins in occiput, spreads upwards and settles over right eye.
Headache with nausea and vomiting, followed by flushes of heat, extending from the head to the stomach.
Nasal polypi.
Red cheeks with burning in ears; with cough.
Vomiting of bitter water; of sour acrid fluids, of ingesta, or worms, preceded by anxiety. Headache better after vomiting, with prostration.
Dry cough with considerable tickling in throat pit and a crawling sensation, extending down beneath the sternum.
Whooping cough.
Asthmatic bronchitis; severe dyspnoea.
Rust coloured expectoration.
Pneumonia; better lying on back.
Rheumatism of right shoulder; worse at night, cannot raise arm.
Right sided brachalgia; lameness and numbness of right arm.
Hay fever form pollen grains.
Lassitude, not inclined to make any mental exertion
Worse in damp weather.

Modalities: Worse from sweets, right side, motion, touch, Better acids, sleep, darknes

Dosage : 200th or higher.

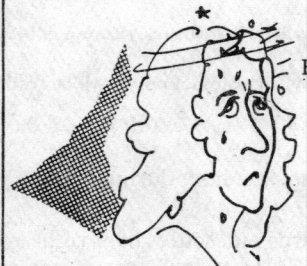

HEADACHE, NAUSEA AND VERTIGO

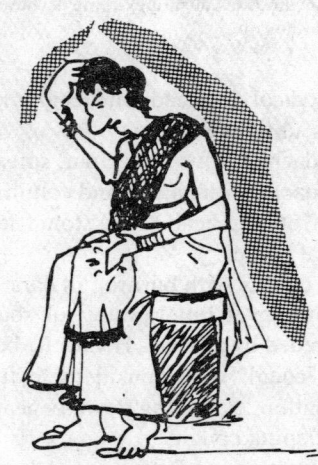

TIRED WITH BEARING DOWN PAINS

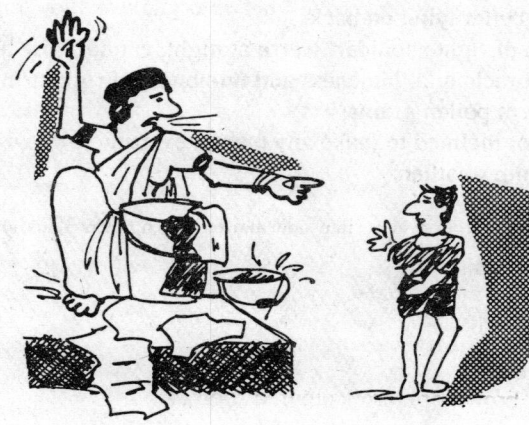

IRRITABLE - INDIFFERENT - APATHETIC TO EVERYTHING.

SEPIA

Common name cuttle fish N.O.Cephalopoda. Trituration of dried liquid contained in the ink bag.

Pathogenetic sphere of action
- The venous circulatory system and portal system causing hepatic engorgement and pelvic congestion.
- The connective tissues causing visceral ptosis and a tendency to varicose veins and haemorrhoids.
- The nervous system causing depression.

Very irritable. Indifferent. Apathatic.
Very indifferent even to her own family, her husband, her children and to those she loved best.
Uneasiness in the presence of strangers.
Headache right sided, with aversion to food, every morning with nausea, vertigo and epistaxis; better after meals.
Ptosis, great falling of hair.
Yellow spots on face and a yellow saddle across the upper part of the cheeks and the nose. Blemishes on face.
Sensitive to noise, music, odors.
Increased hunger or no appetite.
Aversion to food, meat and fat.
Milk causes diarrhoea.
Smell of cooking food nauseats.
Sensation of bearing down of all pelvic organs, as though the contents would escape out.
Constipation, during pregnancy.
Sensation of ball, in anus not relieved by stools.
Nocturnal enuresis; the bed is wet almost as soon as the child goes to sleep.
Prolapsus of uterus, of vagina, with constipation.
Yellowish leucorrhoeal discharge. Metrorrhagia. Amenorrhoea.
Sudden hot flushes at climactric with momentary sweat, weakness and tendency to faint.
Spasmodic cough; worse night.
Pain in back across hips; when stooping; better pressing back against something hard.
A short walk fatigues much.
Sudden prostration and faintness.
Herpes circinates. Ring worm. Profuse night sweat.
Intertrigo; brown or claret coloured spots.

Modalities: Worse forenoons and evenings, washing, laundry work, dampness, leftside, after sweat, cold air, before thunderstorm.Better by exercise, pressure, warmth of bed, hot applications, drawing limbs up, cold bathing, after sleep.

Dosage : 200th 3 doses a day for a considerable period.

144

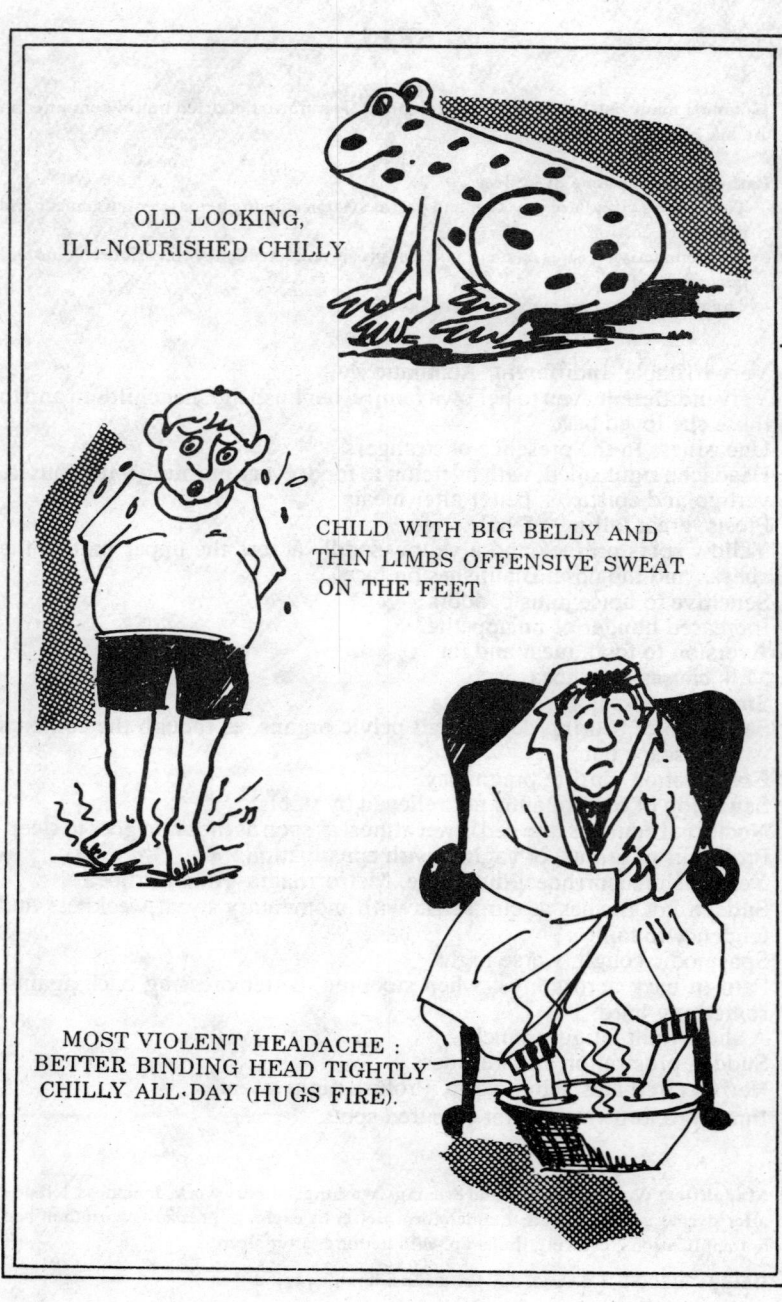

OLD LOOKING,
ILL-NOURISHED CHILLY

CHILD WITH BIG BELLY AND
THIN LIMBS OFFENSIVE SWEAT
ON THE FEET

MOST VIOLENT HEADACHE :
BETTER BINDING HEAD TIGHTLY
CHILLY ALL·DAY (HUGS FIRE).

SILICEA

Silicea terra. Pure flint. Silicion dioxide S_1O_2. Trituration of pure, precipitated silica.

Pathogenetic sphere of action
- The nutrition
- The nervous system
- On suppurative phenomena causing either elimination of pus or foreign bodies thus preventing suppuration.

Extremely chilly; Lack of vital heat; must wrap up, especially head.
Sensitive to noise; Great difficulty in fixing the attention.
Though difficult, always busy in searching for pins.
Headache rising from nape of neck to vertex; As if head would burst; relieved by warm wrapping up of the head.
Sensation of hair lying on the tongue.
Moisture in the anus.
Haemorrhoids painfully sensitive.
Constipation, stool hard, nodular like clay stones.
Fissure ani and fistula in ano.
Expectoration thick, lumpy, yellow.
Purulent expectoration.
Stiffness of nape of neck, with headache.
Limbs falls asleep at night.
Finger nails rough and yellow. Whitlow.
Offensive perspiration on the soles, the parts become sore when walking.
Great weariness and weakness.
Complaints worse at new moon by motion.
Small wound heal with difficulty and easily suppurate.
Several boils come out on whole body.
Profuse offensive perspiration at night.
Weak, punny children not from lack of nourishment but from defective assimilation.
Sweaty headed, over sensitive, imperfectly nourished children.
Big belly; face, old looking.
Learns to walk late.
Stool partly protrude and then recedes back.
Aversion to mother's milk and vomits it easily.

Modalities: Worse new moon, in morning, from washing, during menses, uncovering, lying down, damp, lying on left side, cold. Better warmth, wrapping up head, summer, in wet humid weather.

Dosage : 30th or higher.

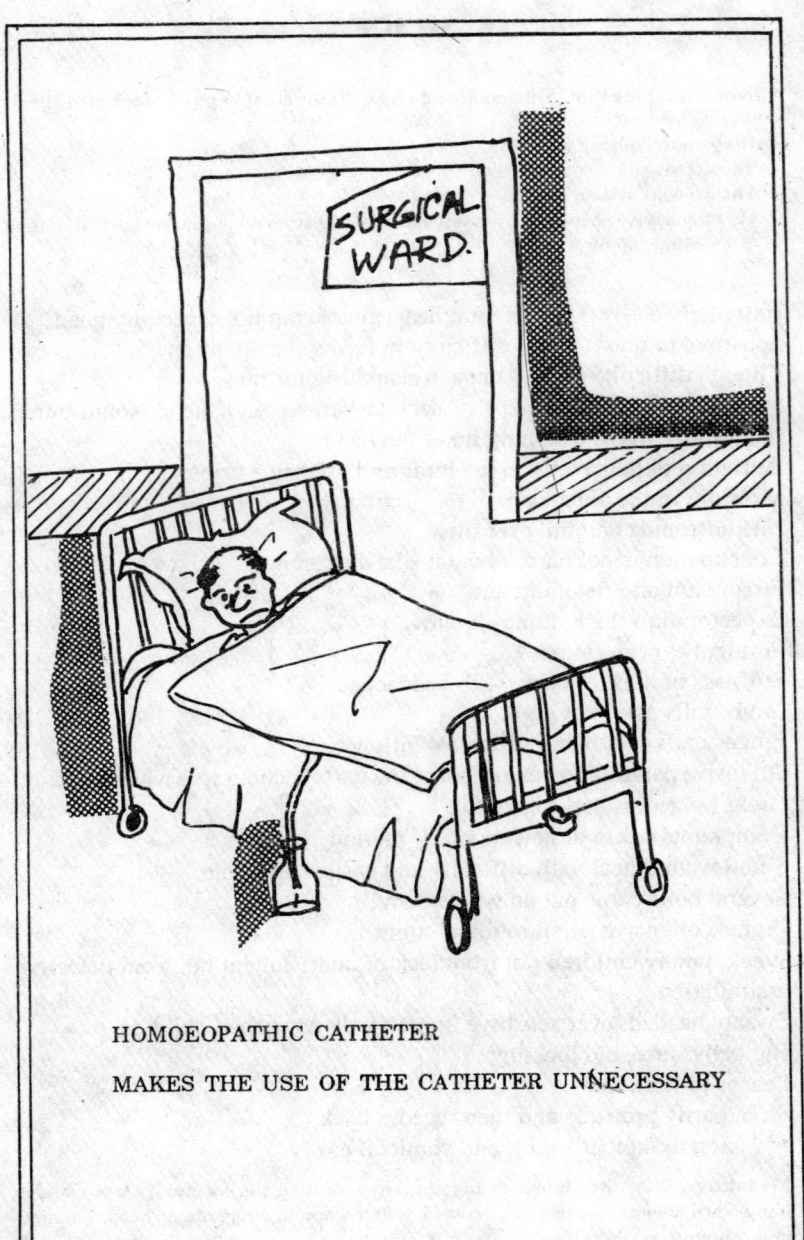

HOMOEOPATHIC CATHETER

MAKES THE USE OF THE CATHETER UNNECESSARY

SOLIDAGO VIRGA

Solidago virgaurea. golden rod.N.O. compositae. Tincture of whole fresh plant. Tincture of flowers.

Pathogenetic sphere of action
- The hepato renal system causing drainage.
- There is painful sensitivity to pressure over both costolumbar regions.
- Prostate-Hypertrophy, Retention of urine.

Repeated cold of tuberculosis, feeling of weakness.

Bronchitis; cough with much purulent expectoration. Haemoptysis with dyspnoea.

Kidneys sensitive to pressure. Glomerulonephritis.

Fibroid tumours.

Benign hyperplasia of prostate.

Difficult, albuminous, scanty, clear and offensive urine.

It makes the use of Catheter unnecessary in case of retention and retention with over flow.

Blotches especially on lower extremeties, itching.

Modalities : Throat infection, chill, alcohol. Better profuse urination.

Dosage : 3x in respiratory ailments. Q for prostate and renal, ursinary condition.

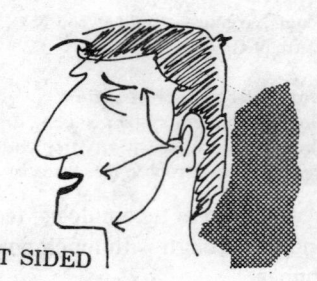

TRIGEMINAL NEURALGIA; LEFT SIDED

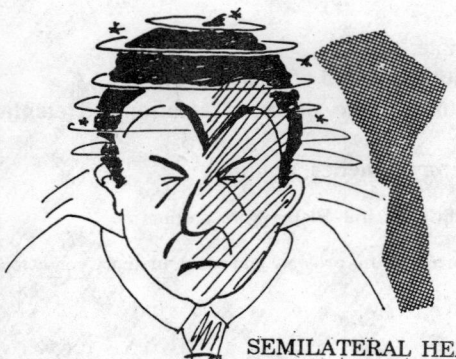

SEMILATERAL HEADACHE; LEFT SIDED

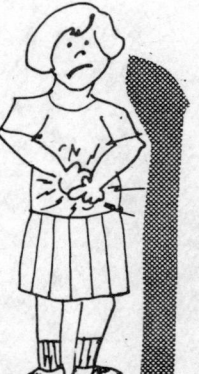

PAIN AROUND NAVEL (WORMS)

SPIGELIA

Spigelia anthelmia. Demerara Pink root. N.O. Loganiaceae.Tincture of dried herb.

Pathogenetic sphere of action
- The nervous system causing neuralgia particularly in trigeminal and intercostal nerves.
- The heart causing violent palpitations.

Very sensitive to touch.

Parts feel chilly send shudder through frame.

Pain beneath frontal eminence and temples extending to eyes.

Eyes feel too large; pressive pain on turning then. Severe pain in and around eyes extending deep into socket.

Discharge through posterior nares chronic catarrah with post nasal dropping of bland mucus.

Foul odour from mouth.

Prosopalgia involving eye, zygoma, cheek, teeth, temple worse stooping, touch, from morning until sunset.

Dyspnoea must lie on right side with head high.

Modalities: Worse touch, motion, noise, turning, washing concussion. Better lying on right side with head high, inspiring.

Dosage : 200th or higher few doses.

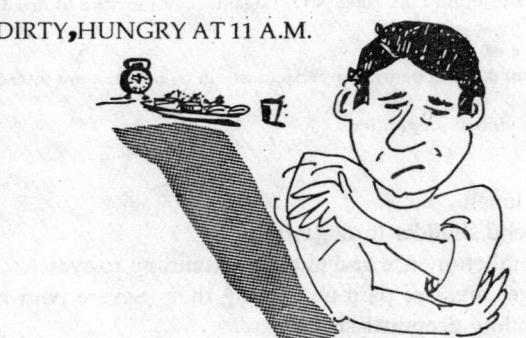

DIRTY, HUNGRY AT 11 A.M.

– ITCHING AND REDNESS
(PRONE TO SKIN AFFECTIONS)

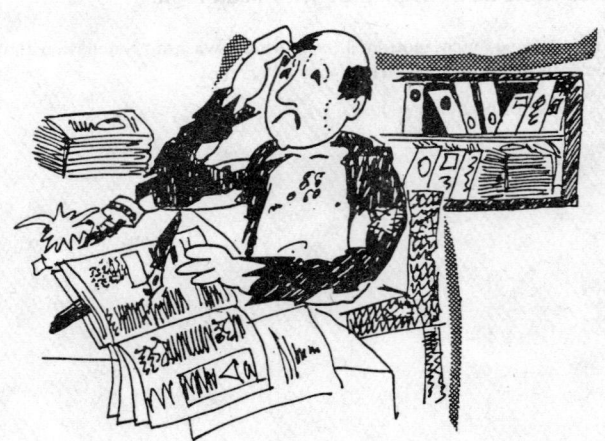

RAGGED PHILOSOPHER.

SULPHUR

Brimstone. sublied sulphur S.(A.W. 31.98). Trituration of "flowers of sulphur"
A saturatued solution of sulphur in absolute alcohol constitutes the tincture.

Pathogenetic sphere of action
- Action in centri fugal from with in outward.
- Skin-producing heat and buring.
- Complaints that relapses.

Lean, thin, stoop shouldered persons.

Dirty, Filthy, prone to skin infections.

Foolish happiness and pride, thinks himself in possession of beautiful things; even rags seem beautiful. Disclined to work, talk or move.

Melancholia; Dwelling on religious or philosophic speculations.

Too lazy to rouse himself up, and too unhappy to live.

Dread of being washed, especially in children.

Head feels hot on top. Itching pimples on fore head.

Dimness of vision; as from a fog, with headache. Painful, hot lachrymation. Otitis.

Frequent sneezing with offensive discharge.

Apthae. Bright redness of lips burns, cracked and dry. Toothache in open air.

Appetite excessive, feeling of faintness at 11 a.m. Drinks much, but eats little.

Desires sweets; diseases from eating sweets, candy etc.

Abdomen bloated with wind. Flatus horribly offensive.

Portal stasis; Haemorrhoids, moist, itching.

Sudden call to stool on waking in morning. Diarrhoea after midnight.

Dysentery; worse early morning. Burning in anus, and urethra.

Hot flushes at climacteric period.

Oppression of chest, feels suffocated; wants doors and windows open.

Palpitation with sharp stitches in precordial region.

Pain in small of back; could not walk erect, was obliged to walk, bent over.

Rheumatic pain in shoulder, expecially in left.

Burning in soles on stepping, after sitting a long time.

Sleep disturbed; wakes up at 3, 4 or 5 a.m.

Complaints from suppressed eruptions. Discharges, acrid, excoriating the skin.

Complaints continually relapsing.

Itching all over the body. Spots painful after itching, with turning. Boils

Modalities: Worse at rest, standing, in bed, washing, morning, alcohol. Better, dry, warm, weather, lying on rt. side.

Dosage : Act in all potencies. 30th or 200th to start with.

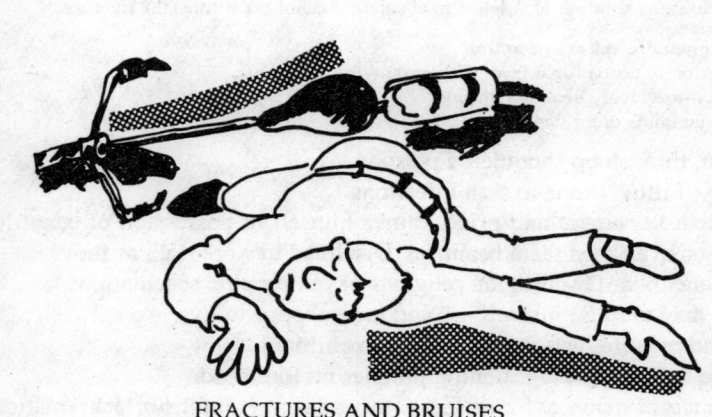

FRACTURES AND BRUISES

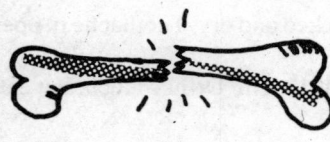

"BONE SET" HERB.

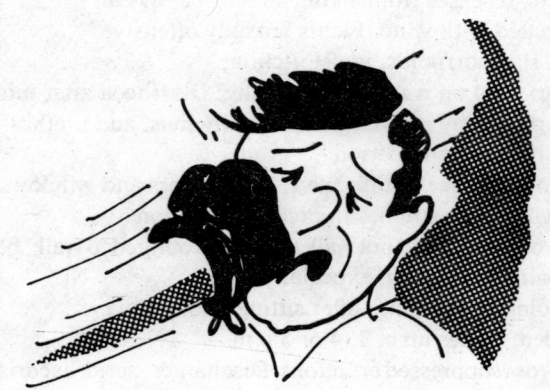

BLOWS: ESPECIALLY AROUND EYES

SYMPHYTUM

Commonly called symphytum officinale Common name Bone set. Healing Herb, N.O. Boraginaceae.Tincture of fresh root stock collected before flowering and in autumn. Tincture of fresh plant.

Pathogenetic sphere of action
- The bones and periosteum.

Bone lesions and fractures.
Bones fails to unite, facilitates union.
Favours production of callus.
Inflammation of bones, diseased spinous processes.
Irritability of bones, at point of fracture; cancer of bone.
Peculiar pain in periosteum after wound has healed.
Gun shot wounds.
Psoas abscess

Modalities : Worse mal nutrition.

Dosage : 30th few doeses daily for a considerable period.

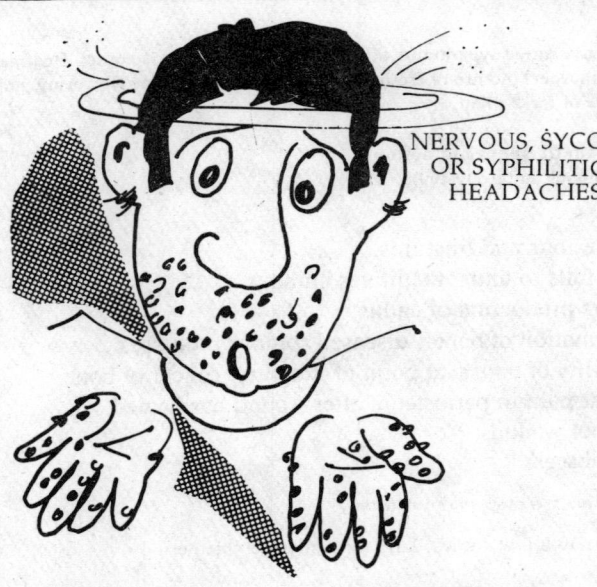

NERVOUS, SYCOTIC
OR SYPHILITIC
HEADACHES

"WARTS", HAIRS DRY AND FALLING OUT

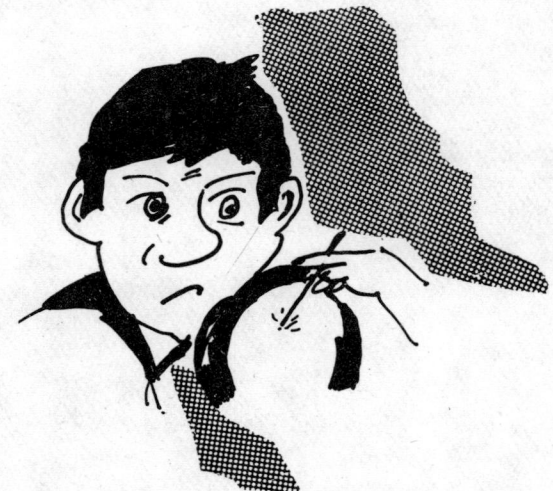

AILMENTS FOLLOWING VACCINATION "VACCINOSIS":

THUJA OCCIDENTALIS

Arbor vitae.N.O.Coniferae. Tincture of fresh green twigs.

Pathogenetic sphere of action
- Genito urinary organs causing inflammation, catarrah, ulcers.
- The skin causing papulo-vesiculo-pustular eruptions.
- The lymphatic system. causing hypertrophy of lymphoid organs.
- The nervous system causing neuralgia and a state of indolence and nervousness with a tendency to have obsessions.

Great ANTI SYCOTIC REMEDY for hydrogenoid constitutions.
Cases with history of snake bite, vaccinations.
Makes mistakes in reading with writing.
Prolonged thinking about the merest trifles.
Fixed ideas, as if the body were brittle and would easily break; when walking, as if legs were made of wood; as if living animal were in abdomen.
Feels as if under the influence of superior power.
Sleeplesness; dreams of falling from a height, of dead people etc.
Nervous, sycotic or syphilitic headache; pain as if pierced by a nail; left sided headache. White scaly dandruff; hair dry and falling out.
Ciliary neuralgia. Chronic otitis with purulent discharge. Eye styes and tarsal tumours.
Aversion to fresh meat and potatoes.
All symptoms worse by ONIONS.
Flatulent distension, protruding here and there.
Haemorrhoids swollen; burning pain in anus.
Anus fissured with warts, condylomata.
Gonorrhoea; scalding pain in urethra when urinating.
Inflammation of urethra with greenish discharge.
Prostatic enlargement. Chronic induration of testicles.
Ovaritis; worse left side.
Asthma in children.
Warts, polypi, tubercles. Ulcers especially in ano - genital regions.
Warts, condylomata, large, seedy, pedenculated.
Brown spots on hands and arms.
Eruptions only on covered parts.
Sweat only on uncovered parts.

Modalities: Worse at night. from heat of bed. at 3 a.m., and 3 p.m., from cold. damp air. after breakfast. fat. coffee. vaccination. Better left side. while drawing up a limb.

Dosage : 200th to start the case. Repeatedly for warts.

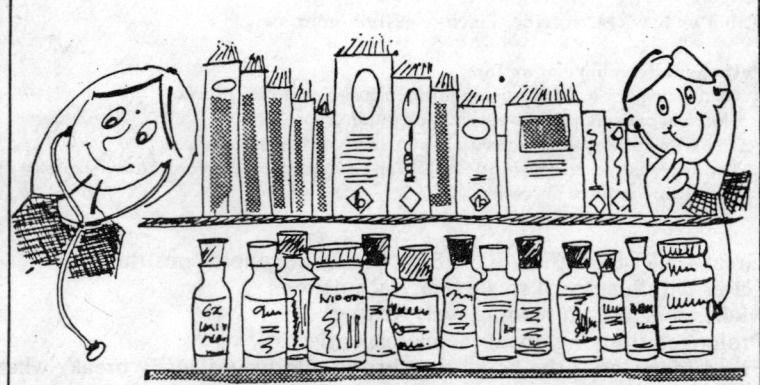

WELL SELECTED REMEDY FAILS TO IMPROVE

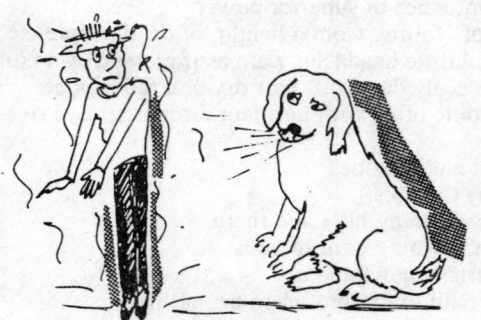

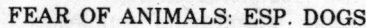

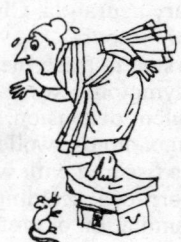

FEAR OF ANIMALS: ESP. DOGS.

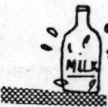 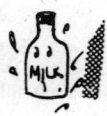

DESIRE COLD MILK

TUBERCULINUM

Tuberculin of koch. A glycerine extract of a pure cultivation of tubercle bacilie liquid attenuations.

Pathogenetic sphere of action
- The respiratory system causing extreme cold sensitivity with a catarrahal condtion-
- Renal, intestines.
- The hepato-digestive system and skin

Depression, melancholia
Nocturnal hallucination; wakes up frightened.
Abuses, use foul language, curse and swear.
Neuralgias in head; as if iron bands around head.
Tubercular meningitis.
Plica polonica, Seborrhic dermatitis, boils with green foetid pus.
Averse to meat, desires cold milk.
Early morning sudden diarrhoea.
There is rapid decrease of vitality with marked weight loss.
Incipient tuberculosis.
When symptoms are constantly changing and well selected remedies fail to improve.
Tendency to catch cold from slightest exposure
Acute articular rheumatism.
Depressed, fear of dogs, animals especially.
Persistent offensive otorrhoea. Perforation in membrana tympani with ragged edges
Benign mammary tumours, dysmenorrhoea, pains increase with the establishments of the flow.
Enlarged tonsils.Longs for cold, fresh air. Bronchopneumonia in children.
Deposits in apex of lungs.
Chronic eczema, intense itching<night. Acne in tuberculers. Psoriasis.
Continous fever, profuse sweat, genral chilliness.

Modalities: Worse motion, music, before a storm, standing,dampness, draught, early morning and after sleep. Better open air.

Dosage : More frequent repetition in acute and children diseases. 30 th. Chronic, non reacting cases 1000 one dose and, wait.

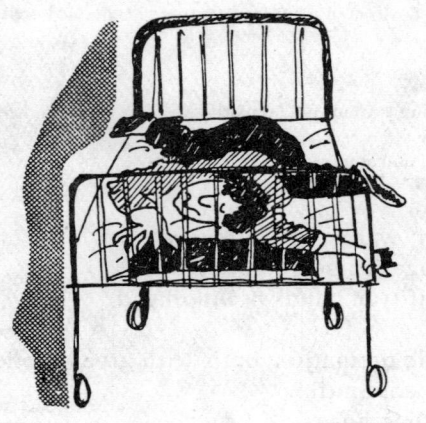

SHOCK

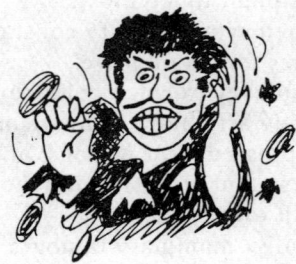

MANIA WITH DESIRE
TO CUT AND TEAR THINGS

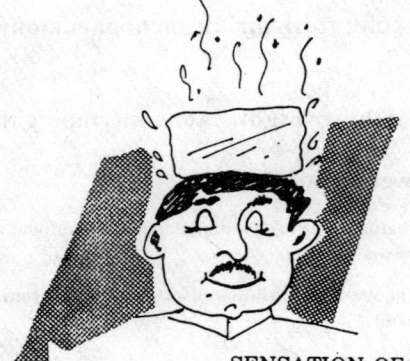

SENSATION OF ICE CAP ON VERTEX

VERATRUM ALBUM

White Hellbore N.O. Melanthaceae.Tincture of root stocks collected early in june before flowering.

Pathogenetic sphere of action
- The digestive tract producing cholera like symptoms.
- The nervous system causing rapid prostration, cramp like manifestations.

Collapse with extreme coldness,blueness and weakness.

Cold perspiration on the forehead.

Vomiting, purging and cramps in extremities.

Profuse, violent retching and vomiting is most characteristic.

"Coprophagia" violent mania alternates with silence and refusal to talk.

Sullen indifference, delusions of impending misfortunes.

Cold sweat on forehead, sensation of a lump of ice on vertex.

Icy coldness of tip of nose of face, face very pale, blue, collapsed and cold.

Thirst for cold water but is vomited as soon as swallowed. Copious vomiting and nausea, aggravated by drinking and least motion.

Cold feeling in stomach and abdomen.

Stools large with much straining until exhausted with cold sweat.

Diarrhoea very painful, watery, copious and forcibly evacuated followed by great prostration.

Dysmenorrhoea with coldness, purging, cold sweat, faints from least exertion.

Cramps in calves.

Skin,blue, cold, clammy, inelastic cold as death.

Chill with extreme coldness and thirst.

Modalities: Worse at night, wet, cold weather. Better walking and warmth.

Dosage : 6th or 30th frequently. 1000 or above in maniacal ailments.

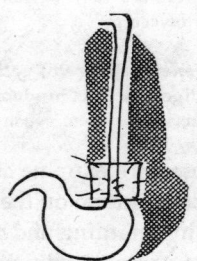

OESOPHAGITIS

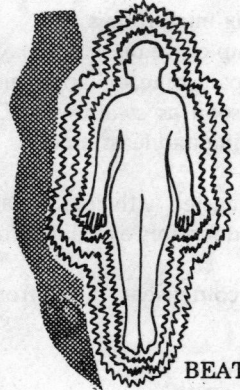

BEATING OF PULSES THROUGHOUT BODY

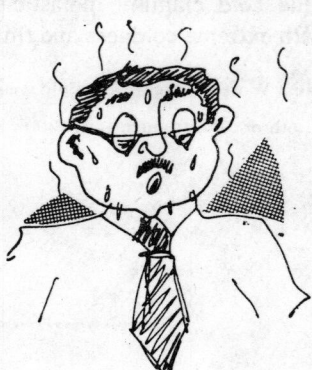

HOT SWEATING

VERATRUM VIRIDE

American white Hellebore. Indian Poke. N.O. Melanthaceae. Tincture of fresh root gathered in autumn.

Pathogenetic sphere of action
- The circulatory system causing congestion.

Bloated livid face.

Oesophagitis.

It will raise the opsonic index against diplococcus pneumonia 70 to 109 per cent.

Head retracted, pupils dilated, double vision

Pain from nape of neck, cannot hold head up

Tongue white or yellow with red streak down the middle.

Hiccough excessive and painful, with spasms of oesophagus.

Croup

Pulse slow, soft, weak, irregular intermittent.

Beating of pulses through out body especially in right thigh.

Acute rheumatism.

Hot sweating.

Modalities : Worse, sun, suppressed imenses. Better, onset of discharges, cold atmosphere.

Dosage : 6th or 30th few doses a day.

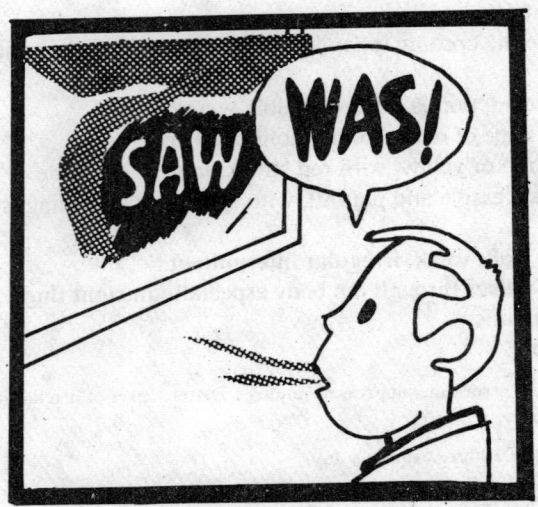

DYSLEXIA; DIFFICULTY WITH WORDS

FORGETS SPELLINGS OF COMMON WORDS;

WRITES LAST LETTERS OF WORDS FIRST

XEROPHYLLUM

Tamal paislily. Basket grass flower. Tincture of flowers.

Pathogenetic sphere of action
- The cerebellum and memory centres
- Congnitive ability.
- The skin.

Dyslexia; difficullty with-words.

It acts in eczematous conditions, poison oak, early typhoid states.

Dull, cannot concentrate mind for study, forgets names,writes last letters of words first

Loss of consciousness.

Misspells common words.

Stuffed, tightness at bridge of nose, acute nasal catarrah.

Eructations sour, offensive an hour after luncheon and dinner. Vomiting at 2 P.M.

Difficulty of retaining urine, dribbling when walking.

Muscular lameness, trembling. Pain in knees.

Erythema with vesication, and intense itching, stinging and burning.

Skin rough and cracked feels like leather.

Dermatitis especially around knees.

Modalities: Worse application of cold water. afternoon. evening. Better application of hot water. morning. moving affected part.

Dosage : 200th infrequent doses.